TAOIST QIGONG

FOR HEALTH AND VITALITY

TAOIST QIGONG

for

HEALTH

and

VITALITY

A Complete Program
of Movement, Meditation,
and Healing Sounds

Sat Chuen Hon

<small>FOREWORD BY PHILIP GLASS</small>

SHAMBHALA · *Boston & London* · *2003*

This book is dedicated with great gratitude to my wife, Janet,

and my daughters, Jimei, Lingji, and Singha.

Shambhala Publications, Inc.
Horticultural Hall
300 Massachusetts Avenue
Boston, Massachusetts 02115
www.shambhala.com

9 8 7 6 5 4 3 2 1

First Edition
Printed in the United States of America

♾ This edition is printed on acid-free paper that meets
the American National Standards Institute z39.48 Standard.

Distributed in the United States by Random House, Inc.,
and in Canada by Random House of Canada Ltd

Library of Congress Cataloging-in-Publication Data
Hon, Sat Chuen.
Taoist qigong for health and vitality: a complete program of
movement, meditation, and healing sounds / Sat Chuen Hon;
foreword by Philip Glass.—1st ed.
p. cm.
ISBN 1-59030-068-8
1. Qi gong. I. Title.
RA781.8.H655 2003
613.7'1—DC21
2003002376

CONTENTS

FOREWORD

T H I S   B O O K   may come as a surprise to many people. It certainly did for me. As a student of Sat Hon's for a number of years, I have concentrated on the longevity practice of Qigong. I've spent many hours with him in his studio in New York City, sometimes arriving a bit early and getting a glimpse of some other class or lesson in process. At his annual Chinese New Year party I have seen fellow students offer demonstrations of their skills. Besides that, I was aware of his training in Traditional Chinese Medicine and acupuncture acquired over many years during his biannual return visits to Beijing. Among his many activities, he conducts a weekly "open door" clinic providing Chinese medicine. In this way I have come to know of the range and depth of his expertise in Qigong, Taiji, and related martial arts forms. He appears to have a near-encyclopedic knowledge of training and practice in his beloved Taoist tradition. Even so, when I first read the manuscript of *Taoist Qigong for Health and Vitality,* I was truly astonished. It presents a healing practice that is largely unknown beyond a small circle of practitioners. Here, in concise and clear language, is a coherent and rich practice combining sound and breath directed toward health and healing.

Furthermore, this book is written with a wealth of personal history and warmth that give insights into Sat Hon's training and practice. Indeed, you can also read the book as a partial autobiography of his own journey on the spiritual path. The work is sprinkled throughout with insights and anecdotes that elucidate and illustrate the spirit of Tao—and not as an academic exercise or translation of a traditional text, but as a seemingly spontaneous reflection by someone living in the practice. The work has gained from this a freshness and joyfulness that place it in a unique class of spiritual literature.

Finally, I would like to touch on another topic that this book indirectly addresses. In Western philosophy and psychology it is referred to as the mind-body problem. The disjunction between body and mind is symptomatic of the pervasive problem many people today have in understanding our common experience of "being in the world." (In serious cases it is expressed as psychotic or autistic behavior.) Traditional healing practice almost always addresses this problem in one way or another. In fact, we can say that healing, in its widest and deepest sense, is precisely about the reunion of mind and body. The great wisdom traditions have considered this issue fundamental to the way we understand our place and how we function in the world. In the Hindu-Buddhist tradition, the union of mind and body is known as the Great Unification. In the Vajrayana practice of Buddhism, it is known as the rainbow body, and this stage of development comes, quite properly, at the end of a long and disciplined practice. This highest state of integration appears in shamanistic and other indigenous traditions as well, either at the end of the practice (as in the Plumed Serpent of the Mayans) or at any point throughout it (as in other Meso-American cultures).

In Taoism—arguably the oldest continuous living tradition apart from the Australian Aboriginal—it appears somewhat differently. Awareness, energy, and body consciousness are considered so fundamental as to allow no delay in addressing them, even at the earliest stages of study. This is amply borne out in the Healing Sounds technique that Master Sat Chuen Hon teaches and bears witness to. From the first page to the last, his narrative is replete with references to an integrated state in which awareness/consciousness and body/energy are meant to function together. Healing, wholeness, and integration become effectively identical in this practice.

The anecdotes and personal history presented here are marvelous. Don't rush through them. Savor them the way you would a bowl of Janet Hon's rice congee soup. You will find some of the best teachings there.

PHILIP GLASS

PREFACE

B Y NATURE, I am lazy. After completing my schooling,
rather than applying for a "serious job," as my mother would
have said, I chose instead just to drift along with the current
of life. It was a decision that I made as a young man in my twenties.
By pure luck, such drifting has led me to the ancient shamanistic
realm of Taoist practices, Qigong and Taiji Quan. Since then, it is
this lazy, at-ease approach that has guided me in my life.

Perhaps I was inspired by my name; it was given to me by a
soothsayer. After gazing into the ether of my future, he gave me the
name Sat Chuen, Stone-Tumbling Stream. My life has been a series
of tumbling acts that flow like meandering streams, stumbling over
different terrains with no discernible goal or purpose.

Similarly, the practice of Qigong and Taoist movements induces
in me an inner sensation like clouds drifting across the halcyon sky.
Sometimes, when I plunge deeply into Taoist practice, I come upon
the still water of nonbecoming, *wu-wei*, a state of utter harmony
where there is neither becoming nor striving. As I gain insight into
the stillness of nonbecoming, this effortless way of moving, my own
movements improve and my energy flows more freely.

Tao is the unfolding of one's spontaneous nature without the im-
position of will. Taoist practices of Qigong and Taiji Quan thrive

within this at-ease, open context of natural spontaneity. The Tao *embraces* the creative principle of life. It holds to the great "mind" of the universe to guide our daily actions. As you begin to practice the Healing Sounds Qigong, keep yourself as much at ease as possible.

This book is derived from a series of lectures that I have presented on the Taoist Six Healing Sounds, which I lightheartedly refer to as "Sing-Along Qigong."

Probably I would not have done anything further with the lectures if it had not been for my student Chris Jurak, who volunteered to transcribe and edit them.

I view this book as the fruition of the labor of a community that includes my family—my wife, Janet, and my three girls, Jimei, Lingji, and Singha—as well as my family of students, who urged me to go deeper into Taoist practice. I would like to express my gratitude to the following individuals who have greatly contributed to the creation of this book and who made it a truly cooperative effort: Philip Glass for his generosity in writing the foreword and for serving as my guide in the labyrinthine world of publishing; Ilana Storace for being the photographer as well as the model for some of the photographs; Sue Terry, Chris Jurak, Beth Frankl, and Mark Magill for editing the book; and Chris Jurak for taking the early storyboard photographs and designing the initial layout. Andrew and Ann Sterman, Ilana Storace, and Erva Zuckerman also contributed suggestions for the book. I am grateful for the generosity of Rudy Wurlitzer, who hand-delivered the manuscript to Sam Bercholz. Mr. Bercholz gave the manuscript its first nourishment along its meandering path to becoming a book. I would also like to thank Carole Corcoran for her legal advice and guidance on contractual matters.

Finally, readers should exercise caution in following the Qigong exercises. As with any sort of physical or mental practice, one should progress slowly. And if any discomfort is felt doing any of the following activities, it is strongly recommended that readers seek medical advice and competent guidance in their practices.

May the merits of this book return to all sentient beings.

PRONUNCIATION GUIDE

THROUGH THE MILLENNIA, the Chinese language has gone through many changes, and many words are spoken with different intonations and dialects. This linguistic variation gives rise to different pronunciations of the Healing Sounds. The following is a phonetic guide to the sounds of the Chinese terms used in this book. For an audio recording of the Healing Sounds, you can log on to the *www.dantao.com* website. A sound is better than a thousand words.

Phonetic Pinyin	English phonetic equivalent
Chu	Chu
Fu	Fu
Hey	Hei
Ho	Huo
Qi	Chi
Qigong	Chi Kung
Xi	Hsi
Xu	Hsü
Tao	Dao

TAOIST QIGONG

FOR HEALTH AND VITALITY

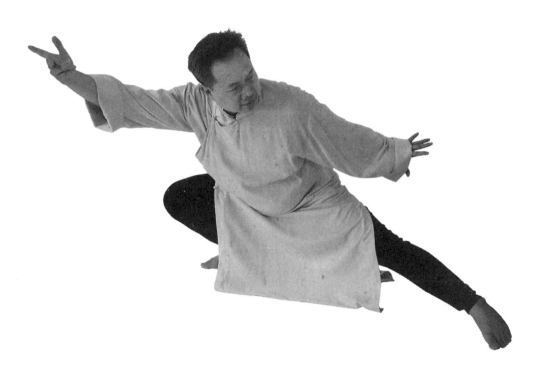

Dragon Humming

SONG OF THE SHAMANS

THE HUMMING FROM ANTIQUITY
Singing of a Stone

Seeking out an old hermit,
I climb the snowy peak to find his thatched hut empty.
As I descend empty hearted,
Suddenly, a wild singing, like murmurs of a dragon,
Echoes from the cloud-shrouded peak.

—based on a Tang Taoist tale (500 C.E.)

History and Development of Taoist Healing Sounds Qigong

Since the beginning of time, shamans would wrap their bodies in bearskin, don an antler headpiece, and sing behind an eagle-beak mask; they would sway in a slow, lumbering gait while whistling piercing trills on a bone flute and calling to the Great Spirit. This is the origin of Taoist Healing Sounds, a wild, mystical singing from the beginning of time. Even in the present day, dwelling deep in some bamboo grottos, Taoist hermits still greet and sing to each other, wailing across valleys like lemurs.

In time, the Healing Sounds, which strengthen and vitalize one's life force, became integrated into internal alchemical practice. The objective of internal alchemy is to transform transitory, mortal life into immortality. This parallels the process of mineral alchemy, which has the similar objective of transmuting mutable lead into immutable gold. Both internal and mineral alchemy express the grand vision of Taoism: that everything and everyone are moving toward a final state of perfection and completion—from lead to gold, from mortality to immortality.

In comparison, during the Middle Ages in Europe, Western alchemists focused primarily on mineral alchemy, mainly on how to turn any object into gold. Hence, the *chem* in *alchemy* still retained its Chinese root meaning "gold." At its core, *al-chemy* is still the art of transmuting objects into gold.

Later, alchemy was dismissed by scientists as superstitious and obsolete. They severed their ties with alchemy by lopping off the prefix *al-* and retaining only the root, chemical aspect of the science. Nevertheless, modern chemistry still owes a great debt to the earlier art of alchemy.

Alchemy was not revisited by any serious scientist in the West until the early twentieth century, when it was reexamined by the eminent psychologist Carl Jung in his psychological writings. Jung discovered that in alchemical symbolism lay the foundation of humans' deep consciousness of fundamental archetypes. These archetypes gave him great insight into the deeper layers of the human psyche: that the symbols of alchemy dwell in our collective unconscious. However, Jung dealt primarily with the psychological archetypes in alchemy, not with its "magical" aspects of physical transformation.

On the other hand, the study of Taoist alchemy as a living art requires a direct, one-to-one transmission from teacher to disciple. Even though thousands of alchemical texts and books exist, beginners must still rely on a personal guide to lead them through the labyrinth of Taoist alchemy. Without such a living guide, relying solely on the surface meaning of alchemical texts is dangerous. This is especially true when dealing with information culled from original Taoist texts, because most of the information they present is encoded. In other words, much of the Taoist classics were written in intentionally ambiguous terms, using colorful symbolism—"the lunar child swallows the vermilion phoenix"—that serves only as an encryption of the real meaning. Therefore, the true practice is passed orally from teacher to disciple, "from mouth to ear," as my teacher would fondly say. Hence, written texts can serve as a reference that must be decoded. (In the above example, the lunar boy represents shiny liquid, mercury. His swallowing the vermilion phoenix can be interpreted as the mercury dissolving the red cinnabar crystals. A further layer of meaning can also be understood as letting one's luminous awareness dissolve the egotistic fire of the heart.)

So one must approach the study of Taoist alchemy with caution; many English translations of Taoist texts exist today, but they should serve only as reference guides for beginners, not as "how-to manuals." But finding a living Taoist master is harder than catching sight of a snow leopard. Many Taoist teachers were persecuted and tortured during the endless cycles of political upheaval and mass purges in Communist China. As I write this book, it is still going on. Therefore, in mainland China today, only a handful of Taoist teachers survive to carry on the ancient tradition of Taoist alchemy—which has a modern name, Qigong.

Within this historical context, anyone who had the good fortune to know the Taoist art is propelled by a sense of urgency and grave responsibility to pass on this ancient treasure. The Taoist Healing Sounds in their simplicity embody all the basic shamanistic and alchemical elements: breath, mudra, movements, and totemic sounds. Thus, the Healing Sounds can serve as a safe haven for beginners to take their first step in Taoist Qigong, as well as an effective key for adepts to unlock and gain entry into the mystery of alchemy.

It is said that a thousand-mile journey starts with a single step. But make sure that this first step is in the right direction. If it is not, then all the steps that follow are for naught.

Now, let's take our first step.

My own journey of healing started with my family. In the summer of 1950 in Guangzhou, China, my mother was cooling off in an alley outside our house. It was an especially hot and humid night, and all the neighbors were outside, cooling themselves and chatting. Somehow, amid the droning voices and the tangy fragrance of jasmine, my mother fell asleep on a small army cot with her newborn son under the full moon. As the night started to cool, she was woken abruptly by the wailing of her baby. Hurriedly, she took him back into the house, but it was too late. He had caught a cold from the chill. By the next day, his body started to burn with fever. As she pressed her lips to his forehead, she felt the scorching, searing heat. She knew then that it was a very dangerous fever.

This was a difficult period for our family. My father's business had collapsed after World War II. We were branded as landlords; everything was taken away, and our house was our only remaining possession. Lacking money to see a doctor, my mother tried toughing it out, hoping that the baby's fever would run its course in a few days. But the fever continued to spike higher.

In desperation, she swallowed her pride and went to the local charity organization, which dispensed herbs. But even with the prescribed herbs, the baby's fever remained high. By the third week, he had become too weak even to cry. Once in a while, he would give out a fitful, pitiful whimper, his fists balled up in pain.

Finally, my mother scraped together enough money to see a Chinese doctor. But the doctor could not find any pulse at the baby's wrist; only at his ankles was there still some weak pulse. The doctor halfheartedly wrote out a prescription and told my mother to pray for the best.

Racked with despair, my mother walked aimlessly along the bank of the Pearl River. An old woman noticed her crying and the lifeless baby in her arms.

"Young miss, what's the matter with your baby?" the old woman asked.

My mother told her the whole story, how even the doctor had given up hope.

"Why don't you try having your baby adopted by the Carp Goddess? Maybe some evil spirit is possessing him."

As a last-ditch effort, my mother took the baby to the Carp Goddess Temple. It was a small provincial temple, and on the altar was just a single statue of the Carp Goddess riding the back of a dragon. Bundles of incense in a bronze urn wafted a musky fragrance in the dimly lit hall. Next to the altar, a small old woman was kneeling on the wooden prayer platform. She was the abbess and the sole caretaker of the temple. My mother told the abbess her wish to have her son adopted by the Carp Goddess.

Chanting strange incantations, the abbess carefully wrapped a yellow paper charm with unfamiliar script on the baby's wrists. Taking some water from a glass vase at the feet of the Carp Goddess, she sprinkled his wrists. Suddenly, three long, dark, bony finger marks appeared on both his wrists, as if something or someone was trying to choke the baby's life force.

"Ah, here's the problem. Your baby must have caught some evil spirit. Let the Carp Goddess claim him as her godchild, and then the dark spirit will leave."

Thunderstruck, my mother suddenly recalled that on the night she had fallen asleep outside, she had seen a shadowy figure standing at the doorway before she went back into the house. She had blamed the shadow on the maid's careless way of drying the laundry on the balcony, but the maid had pointed out that no clothes had been hung to dry that night. Later, my mother discovered that Japanese soldiers had shot and killed a fugitive in the alleyway during World War II.

After a simple ceremony of lighting three red candles and nine sticks of incense, my brother was adopted by the Carp Goddess. No evil spirit would dare to harm him now.

Confidence and hope bloomed in my mother's heart. She gave her son the herbal prescription, and, for the first time in three weeks, the baby fell into a deep sleep. Within a week, he recovered.

Afterward, my brother was forbidden to ever eat carp.

This story reflects the spiritual influence in Chinese Medicine. From the beginning of time, healing was steeped in the shamanistic rituals that tap into the power of the divine spirits of animals, rocks, and natural objects. *The Yellow Emperor's Classic on Internal Medicine*, one of the oldest medical texts in China, states that in olden times, people lived very simply and could expel their sickness with the simple healing *juyui* shamanistic dance. But in the ensuing times of decadence, people needed more complex medical treatments.

My family's healing story illustrates the multifaceted nature of healing and medicine, integrating both the use of medicinal herbs and the spiritual rituals of totems. The spirit of indigenous shamanism is still very much alive in contemporary Chinese culture.

Beginnings of Chinese Medicine

The Yellow Emperor (2697 B.C.E.?–2599 B.C.E.) is a legendary and pivotal figure in ancient Chinese history. He served the dual roles of divine ruler, who was called the Son of Heaven, and founder of Chinese medicinal healing. The Yellow Emperor had learned from the great Taoist hermits Kuang Shen Tze (Vast Numinous Exalted Elder) and Jade Maiden. Kuang Shen Tze taught him the use of herbs and acupuncture in healing, while Jade Maiden showed him the way of sexual cultivation to achieve health and healing, Taoist tantric healing.[1] Afterward, the Yellow Emperor dictated these teachings to his ministers in order to educate the people, and they were later compiled into *The Yellow Emperor's Classic on Internal Medicine*. This canonical text is still used in China as a major source in teaching Traditional Chinese Medicine (TCM).

After a golden reign of almost a hundred years, during which the Yellow Emperor's queen, Lunar Moth, discovered the art of silk weaving and his marquis established the first coherent Chinese dictionary, the Yellow Emperor retired to begin his cultivation of immortality. After nine years, he succeeded in creating his Immortal Elixir. The emperor bade farewell to his court and ascended to the peak of Tai Shan Mountain. Waiting for him there to assist his ascension to heaven was a dragon. As the emperor rode the dragon to heaven, some of his courtesans clung to its tail, but they were shaken off and left behind. This is the eternal lesson of life: One cannot ride on the coattail of another's immortal accomplishment. The Immortal Elixir has to be self-generated.

This legend of the Yellow Emperor symbolizes the dual development of medical science and shamanism. These two lineages intertwine like two serpents, giving rise to the later developments of Taoist healing practice and alchemy.

In the historical arena, the First Emperor, Qin Shihuangdi (r. 221–206 B.C.E.), who conquered the other seven kingdoms and unified China into a single empire, tried to emulate the mythic Yellow Emperor's achievement of immortality. This was no surprise. After one has conquered the world, the only remaining goal is immortality. Initially, the Qin emperor sent five hundred boys and girls accompanied by a Taoist master out on the eastern seas to search for the Immortal Elixir. Unfortunately, they never returned. After several failed attempts at attaining immortality, the Qin emperor journeyed to Tai Shan Mountain in order to reenact the Yellow Emperor's heavenly ascension. He had secretly hoped to experience a profound transformation at the peak of Tai Shan Mountain, perhaps even to meet a few immortals. But other than being soaked by a sudden downpour, the emperor came away empty-handed. Afterward, heartbroken, the Qin emperor turned his attention to more mundane projects, including building the Great Wall of China and his vast underworld paradise. It took almost twenty years to complete both projects, and they have become an enduring legacy. His underground paradise later became a repository of archaeological treasures. His tomb was filled with an army of clay soldiers, riders, and alchemical texts. The First Emperor died at the age of fifty-two and his empire lasted for only ten more years after his death. But the search for immortality became the overriding aspiration of all the emperors who succeeded him.

In one of the alchemical texts of Taoist Healing Sounds unearthed from his tomb, fragments clearly showed drawn figures assuming different Qigong postures, along with inscriptions of different sounds to heal sickness. These fragments are some of the earliest evidence that sounds were used to heal illness. Other indications can be found in the writings of ChuangTze (250 B.C.E.), for example: "in the cultivation of life, some people exhale with the sound of CHU and inhale with the sound of HEY to stimulate the flow of their Qi/energy."[2]

Most spiritual practices in China integrate the Healing Sounds as an integral component. During the later development of Buddhism, the Healing Sounds were incorporated as part of the Ten-tai Buddhist sect's meditative process of calming the mind: "if a meditator should ever feel an overwhelming sensation of heat burning inside the body, he should open his mouth and exhale with the sound of HO until the heat is dissipated."[3] And the Ming dynasty acupuncture encyclopedia, *The Complete Work on Acupuncture,* recommended the use of Healing Sounds for the acupuncturist to harmonize his or her own qi before treating patients: "if an acupuncturist can center his/her qi with the Six Healing Sounds, the patient's recovery will be sooner and the treatment will be more energetically beneficial."[4]

In traditional Chinese healing, the state of the healer's qi/energy is essential, especially for the acupuncturist. The insertion of needles in the patient conducts the qi from doctor to patient and vice versa. Practicing the Healing Sounds, the healer can cleanse his or her own energy and detoxify the backflow of the patient's pathogenic qi. During my training at the Guangzhou University of Traditional Chinese Medicine, if an intern was pregnant, she was advised not to treat patients with acupuncture, so as not to deplete her own qi and thereby cause her fetus to be undernourished.

Preliminary Recommendations for Practicing the Healing Sounds

The Healing Sounds Qigong is a safe and effective health practice for almost everyone. I have written this book with the absolute beginner in mind. Fundamentally, the Healing Sounds are meant to be practiced as a general strengthening of one's breath and qi/energetic flow. Even though the Healing Sounds do not need to be practiced in their entirety, beginning students should first read through the entire book, which is arranged according to the organs' natural sequence: liver, heart, spleen, lungs, kidneys, and triple heater. Please do not attempt to treat any specific disease by jumping directly into the most obvious Healing Sounds. For example, someone with a heart ailment is advised against practicing just the Healing Sound for the heart. According to Taoist healing principles, a heart ailment is a state of weakened fire, which may be caused by another organ's dysfunction. In this case, for best results, all six of the Healing Sounds should be practiced.

After completing the book and becoming familiar with the Healing Sounds sequence, you can then choose a particular sound to work on, to unveil the deeper layers of its healing function. As you come to know the sounds, they will unfold for you an intimate knowledge of your body and its workings. After all, the Healing Sounds come from deep within you. You are sounding out from the depth of your being. Listen to the sounds and they will tell you the secrets of your body. After an extended period of practice, you will naturally choose a few particular Healing Sounds as your favorites. This is a very good way of self-discovery. The beginning of the shamanistic journey is the unfolding of our intuitive wisdom.

With daily practice, you will notice the timbre and tonality of the sound. Gradually, as your sinus cavities open, the sounds will acquire a smooth, flutelike quality. A good way to verify your understanding is to tape record your practice sessions, then listen to the tape and check for any strain or tension in the sounds.

The Six Healing Sounds are but a simple gateway to discovering the infinite realm of sound and healing. As you become more sensitive, you will begin to notice how in daily life you constantly make little nonverbal Healing Sounds of your own. Become aware of how those sounds serve to balance you.

In our excessively verbal society, we often neglect the beauty of nonverbal sounds. Music versus noise, words versus nonsense are but the judgment and conditioning of the mind. Dissolve the judgmental and categorizing mind and all noise becomes musical; all nonverbal sounds evoke deep emotions.

During a solitary meditation retreat in a cabin in Vermont, I clearly heard the soothing sound of ocean waves during my midnight sitting. In the morning, I went outside and discovered that the lulling sound of rolling waves I had heard during the night had been traffic noise from smoke-belching trucks careening down the highway. Living in New York City, I had always cringed at noisy traffic. But all sounds can be quite soothing; it depends on one's frame of mind. Similarly, the practice of the Healing Sounds might seem foreign and uncomfortable at first, but with dedicated effort, the sounds will gradually evoke a deep response from our inner body. Our organs will start to resonate with this primal voice of our ancestors. To put a slight twist on the words of Genesis, "In the beginning, before the Word, let there be Sound."

My experience in Vermont reminded me of a faux pas with my teacher. For my teacher's eightieth birthday gift, his students decided to install double-paned windows in his apartment, which perched above the noisy, bustling streets of Chinatown. Sometimes the raw, metallic, grating sounds of traffic were so intrusive that we could hardly hear his words. And since his building was near a fire station, the sirens of fire trucks were a constant disturbance at all hours.

My teacher shook his head and laughed.

"It has taken me ten years of arduous cultivation to transform the sound of the sirens into luminous lines and sinuous curves in my dream state. Thank you for such thoughtfulness, but I have grown fond of the sirens!"

A stanza from the Kuan Yin bodhisattva's meditation came to my mind:

> Entering the stream of sounds, the noise is forgotten and there
> is quiescence.
> In this state, there is neither sound nor silence, movement nor
> stillness.[5]

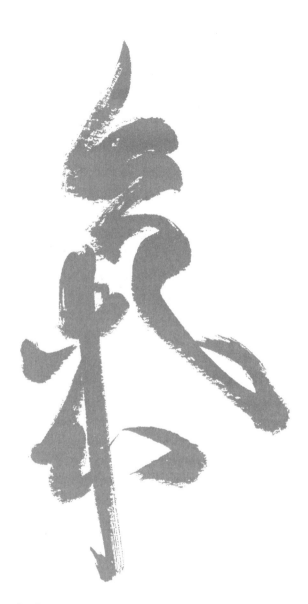

Qi, the Fountain of Life

In Chinese, *qi* (pronounced *chee*) means "breath" and is often translated as "energy." Qi is the life force that constitutes the basic matter of all things. The Chinese pictogram of *qi* presents the image of a wispy vapor rising from fermenting brew, transforming the soup of common grains into an intoxicating broth. This is the dawn of alchemy. The process of fermenting, cooking, and transmuting ordinary matter into spirit and immortality is at the heart of Taoist cultivation.

INTRODUCTION TO THE
TAOIST HEALING SOUNDS

Healing the Body with Sound: I Sing the Body Electric

Let body return to body,
Let mind return to mind,
Let being return to being,
Let breath return to breath,
Let all things return to themselves.
All effort comes to an end.
Awareness emerges like blue sky.
Being aware has no self,
Being aware has no beginning,
Being aware has no time.
In a single moment of awareness,
*   the whole universe is awakened.*

I N T I M E S O F S T R E S S or sickness, we cry out spontaneous sounds that seem to heal our hurt and soothe away our
pain. When we fall down, we cry out, "Ouch." When a mother
holds her baby, she starts to coo. When a patient suffers from a high
fever, a kind of soft, moaning "Hey, hey" is emitted naturally to

release the excessive heat. Being keen observers of nature, Taoists discovered the link between sound and healing. As a result, they mimicked these spontaneous utterances and tempered them into an intricate system of Six Healing Sounds. Traditionally, this practice was referred to as Six Qi Respiration.

To make sense of the therapeutic effect of the Healing Sounds, we have to unearth them from our daily use of sound as only speech. People have long forgotten how to use the primal power of sounds to heal, with the exception of only a few remaining Aboriginal shamans, who still use magical chants in their healing rites to blow away sickness and evil spirits. Sadly, their shaman's craft is in danger of being lost, along with their prehistoric habitats, in the press of modern progress.

Fortunately, two contemporary practices of the Healing Sounds survive. These are the studies of mantras from yoga and the Six Healing Sounds of Taoist alchemy. These two systems are like two streams diverting from a single ancient source; each has developed its own unique and extensive teaching on the interrelationship between organs and Healing Sounds.

The yogic universal mantra AUM consists of three sounds that correspond to the physical body (A), to the soul (U), and to the spirit (M). The mantra affects our being through the sound itself, the meaning of the words, the mental image, and the "spirit" of the mantra.

Paralleling the use of the mantra, the Taoist healing tradition, which dates from 200 B.C.E., expands to encompass the therapeutic and physical effects of sound on the organs. The Six Healing Sounds correspond to the organs in our body: XU to the liver; HO to the heart; FU to the spleen; XI to the lungs; CHU to the kidneys; and HEY to the triple heater. The three major therapeutic effects of the Healing Sounds are to harmonize the organs, open the throat and increase oxygen flow into the bloodstream, and increase qi/energy flow.

The Healing Sounds also have a number of curative effects:

- By using the throat and the esophagus, the Healing Sounds release excessive heat and toxins from the organs.
- Through the shaping of the mouth and tongue, the resonance of the sounds stimulates the internal movement of the organs.
- Through the coordination of physical movements with the sounds, the Healing Sounds enable one to regain one's natural freedom in breathing.

Releasing excessive heat cools the organs, while the vibrations of the sounds stimulate their function. Regaining the spontaneous free breath releases us from the conditioned habit of restricted breathing, increasing the amount of oxygen in our blood.

The Chinese organ system involves more than just the physical organs. For example, the heart is not merely a pump but is regarded as the seat of the consciousness; the heart has a general function in the nervous system. The spleen is responsible not only for the digestive system but also for the control and effect of the body's muscular system. The interrelationship between the organs and the neural, endocrine, musculoskeletal, and immune systems is the distinctive characteristic of TCM. The TCM principle of treating sickness has become widely accepted in the United States and Europe.

The practice of the Six Healing Sounds serves as the trigger point for tweaking the organs into balance and indirectly dealing with the other body systems.

Healing Stories

The following healing stories illustrate the power of sound in healing serious sickness. It is important to note that in both cases the patient was treated by a competent, qualified Qigong healer.

The first case involves two famous Qigong masters living in Beijing, Master Yan and Master Wong. At the time, Master Yan was a young man in his thirties who could heal people by projecting his qi into them. Master Wong was a martial artist with very strong qi who could also heal and relieve his patients' symptoms and sickness by simply touching the affected areas with his palm.

One day, a message was relayed to Master Yan that Master Wong had developed a tumor in his neck. The tumor, being very close to a major artery, was inoperable, and so Master Wong requested Master Yan to come and heal him. When Master Yan heard this, he was slightly surprised because he knew that a common ability of a Qigong master was to use qi projection to shrink tumors, and he wondered why Master Wong could not heal his own tumor.

Master Yan arrived at Master Wong's house and, after having some tea, began his treatment. Placing his palm on Wong's neck, he asked Wong to cry. Being a tough martial artist, Wong replied, "I will never cry! I only bleed!"

So Master Yan started to cry himself, wailing the sounds of "boo-hoo-hoo." He did this for about five minutes, then removed his hand from Master Wong's neck and departed. Master Wong was left wondering at what a strange fellow Master Yan was.

After a week, Master Wong visited Master Yan. During that period, his tumor had shrunk to half its former size.

Master Wong said, "I don't know what you did, but thanks to you, my tumor is reduced by half. Is there any way that I could shrink it completely?"

"Yes," replied Master Yan. "Cry every day until it is totally gone!"

"Why should I cry? That doesn't make any sense. I have never cried in my life, not even when they beat me during the Cultural Revolution. I would not cry out to give them the satisfaction of knowing that I was in pain," Wong shouted.

"Aha," said Master Yan. "That is precisely the cause of your tumor. You have trapped the qi of anger in your neck, and now it has caused the cells to grow and harden into a tumor. When I visited you last time, as soon as I touched your neck I felt this incredible need to weep, to cry out. Since you would not cry, I had to cry for you, or else I myself would have gotten very sick. By crying for you I was able to reduce your choked-up qi by half. Now you have to do the rest yourself. You don't have to cry literally—just do the Healing Sound of HO for five minutes every day, and your tumor will disappear completely."

Master Wong followed Master Yan's instruction, and within a month his tumor had shrunk completely. From this story, one can see that sometimes the Healing Sounds are based on the sounds we make naturally—in this case, the sound of crying—in order to release past trauma.

The second story is my own personal one, which occurred while I was in China doing an internship in a TCM hospital. One day in the obstetrics clinic, we saw a pregnant woman whose fetus had died. She was advised to stay in the hospital and have the fetus removed, but she refused, saying that she would rather deliver the dead fetus naturally. Before she left the clinic, I gave her my number at the hospital complex and told her to give me a call if she had any heavy bleeding.

In the middle of the night, I was woken by the telephone. At the other end was the woman from the clinic, hysterically crying that she was bleeding heavily, nonstop. My first thought was to have her call an ambulance, but she said that an ambulance would not be available till the morning. I realized that by then it might be too late.

So, at three A.M., I pedaled my bicycle furiously to her apartment. Her husband was away on business, and a relative was staying with her. As I walked in, I immediately noticed the tangy smell of blood and panic in the room. The woman had lost a large amount of blood, and when I checked her pulse it was so low that it was almost imperceptible. I was concerned that she might go into shock from losing so much blood.

I decided to try to stop any further bleeding by applying acupuncture to various points on her body. After the insertion of the needles, her bleeding slowed, but then her body started to shake all over. My heart sank, because this was a possible sign that she would go into shock. Desperate, I suddenly remembered what my Qigong master had told me about using the Healing Sounds to help the patient's qi flow. I gently placed my palm on her forehead and started to chant the Healing Sound cycle of XU, HO, FU, XI, CHU, HEY. I must have continued to chant for twenty minutes, and gradually her shaking slowed and finally ceased. Afterward, she fell into a deep sleep. I sat by her bed and kept watch over her for another hour. Suddenly, a pristine clarity infused my whole being that my destiny, my purpose in life, was to use Qigong therapy in healing. Strangely, at that same moment, the woman smiled in her sleep.

I stayed for the rest of the night, sleeping on the sofa. In the morning, my patient delivered the dead fetus naturally. For a moment, in silence, we gazed upon the tiny crimson shape curled up like a small crumbled leaf. Like summer drizzle, my patient started to cry softly. Only then did she finally have the energy to cry.

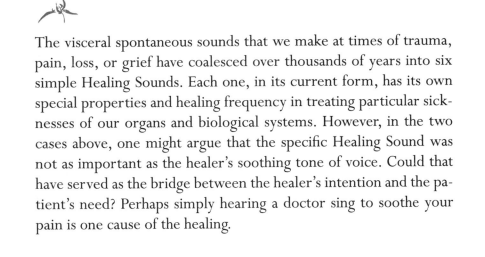

The visceral spontaneous sounds that we make at times of trauma, pain, loss, or grief have coalesced over thousands of years into six simple Healing Sounds. Each one, in its current form, has its own special properties and healing frequency in treating particular sicknesses of our organs and biological systems. However, in the two cases above, one might argue that the specific Healing Sound was not as important as the healer's soothing tone of voice. Could that have served as the bridge between the healer's intention and the patient's need? Perhaps simply hearing a doctor sing to soothe your pain is one cause of the healing.

MACROCOSM AND MICROCOSM

Taoist Concepts of Health and Therapeutics

When a Taoist sees the moon and the sun,
She reflects their light in her eyes.
Seeing the river,
She senses her blood coursing through her veins.

What is outside us—the whole of the universe—
Is mapped within, the small universe of self.

The Cosmic Partnership

The grand concept of Taoist partnership involves the three realms of heaven, human, and earth. In this expansive view, the Taoist sees herself as an integral partner of heaven and earth. Humans are the conduit for the energy between heaven and earth. Without the balancing force of humanity, the world as we know it would collapse. In times of drought, earthquake, and flood, the Taoist looks to the human realm to find the source of the disharmony in the natural environment.

Only in the twenty-first century has humanity come to realize the effect we have in, for example, producing gases that alter the earth's atmosphere. In a computer model of atmospheric drift, an M.I.T. researcher discovered that even the smallest deviation of force (such as a single wingbeat of a butterfly) will, over time, create significant shifts in the weather pattern.

The grand partnership of humanity with the cosmos is the fundamental context of Taoism and all other shamanistic practices. A student once asked me in jest, what would be his contribution to the world if he just sat in a cave gazing at his navel? That would depend on how deeply he gazed at his navel! A single consciousness that achieves liberation and freedom is in perfect fusion with the cosmic order. Even in total physical isolation, such a consciousness will serve as a rare gem, a crystal that gathers the cosmic forces into itself and refracts them out to the whole world.

The Taoist grand view of accomplishment is: Perfect freedom in perfect fusion with the cosmic order.

The Taoist Concept of Health

Health is the free flow of qi/energy between the organs, the meridians, and every pore of the body.
Imagine a healthy tree—its sap must run freely to provide energy to all of its parts—flowers, leaves, and branches.

Sickness is the blockage and stagnation of the qi flow in our body. Imagine a polluted river choked with beer cans and litter—the fish will not survive or even stay healthy in such stagnant water. What is the meaning of qi? There is no literal translation, but qi can be approximated as breath, air, gas, or energy. Qi has its counterpart in yoga as *prana*, in Polynesian and Hawaiin as *mana*, and in Latin as *spiritus*. There are many different types of qi, such as earth qi, sky qi, or food qi. There is also a type of qi specific to the different organs, unique to the functional properties of each. So, in the case of the

Healing Sounds, there is an emphasis on working with the qi of each of the six major organs.

For the Taoist, each organ—the heart, lungs, liver, spleen, kidneys—has three characteristics:

1. Each organ has a special ability. For example, the heart, besides being a simple pump to circulate blood, is also the seat of consciousness and awareness. Many beginning students tend to confuse the physical heart with the Taoist concept of the heart, which encompasses far more than a mere physical organ. In this case, one should regard the heart as part of the visceral nervous system—our "gut feeling" body nervous system. Romeo's heartache for Juliet is in keeping with the Taoist concept of the heart as the seat of consciousness and awareness.
2. Each organ contributes unique substances to the qi stream, our body's overall energetic milieu. For example, the heart contributes fire and warmth to the qi stream. The kidneys contribute the cooling element of water.
3. Each organ asserts a distinctive force in the direction and flow of the energy and nutrients within our body. For example, the lungs have a downward-exerting ability. This force pushes the fluid and blood flow downward. Its movement is contraction and expansion.

The following chart describes some of the organs' major functions, qualities, and movements.

Organ	Special Ability	Unique Substance	Organic Flow
Liver	Detoxifies and cleanses the blood and establishes connectivity between different parts of the body	Contributes tensility and strength, the infrastructure of the body	Asserts an upward flow and causes qi and blood to spread throughout the body

Organ	Special Ability	Unique Substance	Organic Flow
Heart	Is the consciousness, seat of the numinous spirit	Provides internal fire and warmth	Creates spiraling and turning motion in the blood and qi flow
Spleen	Stores nutritional energy and absorbs excessive dampness from the body's internal environments	Transforms food into nutritious substance and qi and passes them to the lungs for distribution	Delivers nutrients upward to the lungs and eliminates wastes downward to the large intestine
Lung	Protects and shields all organs beneath it	Provides coolants and maintains the body's homeostasis	Asserts a downward movement of qi and fluid to the body
Kidney	Stores sexual essence/life force and endocrine hormones	Distributes moisture and life-giving water	Asserts a centripetal, inward-gathering motion on the fluid and qi

The Taoist view is that a healthy person
Will live to one hundred twenty years.
Premature death is due to the degeneration of our organs.
Most people consider themselves old at eighty.
Taoist masters view such premature aging as slow degeneration
    and chronic sickness.

Tracing the Root of Sickness: Avoiding Extremes

What happens when you have too much or too little of one thing? For example, a child who has a real sweet tooth will say, "Gee, two tablespoons of sugar in my hot cocoa is good—so how about ten?"

Does the cocoa taste ten times as good that way? No. It gets too thick. When such oversaturation occurs in the body, according to TCM, there is sickness. When you don't have enough fluid, you have a condition called toxic dryness (your voice may sound sexy, as it becomes low and raspy).

On the other hand, you can have too little of one of the ingredients. I grew up in a family of six; sometimes we had to split a cup of cocoa six ways. We had one spoonful of cocoa for six cups of water. What do you think happened to the cocoa? It was very thin, because there was too much liquid. If such watery dilution happens in the body, it is a condition called toxic dampness. In Western terminology this is called edema, fluid retention. Toxic dampness drains the body's vitality and fire; such a patient will tend to be tired and exhausted. According to the Taoist therapeutic system, the watery dampness has conquered the fire of vitality.

For the Taoist, one of the main causes of damage to our organs is excess. Overconsumption of food, fat, and sugar will generate excessive mucus and phlegm in our blood vessels—like built-up grease in a drain. Eventually, the artery will harden, and blood flow and qi will stagnate. The Chinese call this blockage of phlegm or mucus, and, according to TCM theory, this is a major cause of many cancers. So, for example, when the lungs are in a state of stagnation due to excessive and continuous build-up of phlegm, they start to change into a hard, rocklike substance, and you get what the Chinese call *amjing* (literally, "hardening into rock"), or cancer. Undereating and starvation—the opposite extreme—will obviously weaken the body, making it susceptible to disease and bone loss. Overconsumption of alcoholic drinks—which have a fiery nature—will harden and scorch the liver, which then has to work overtime to neutralize the fire from the bloodstream. Excessive thrills and pleasure damage the heart; pleasure and excitement from either by natural causes or drugs overtax our cardiovascular and nervous systems. Lifestyle excesses will cause the degeneration of our organs' functions and their ability to maintain our health and internal homeostasis. Some examples of results of these excesses include:

- The loss of the organ's unique ability. For example, the heart may become stagnant, causing listlessness and depression.
- The increase or depletion of the organ's substance. When the kidney is drained of its cooling essence, the person becomes overheated and agitated.
- Chaotic and dysfunctional movement of the organs. If the heart goes into chaotic movement, one has cardiac arrhythmia, which can cause serious damage to the heart and possibly result in a heart attack.
- Overheating of the organs. Excessive heating of the liver through too much alcohol consumption leads to hardening of the liver.
- Overcooling of the organs. Overcooling of the stomach from drinking too many cold drinks and eating ice cream will result in general indigestion and inability to absorb nutrients in food.

The following charts delineate some of the major pathologies and dysfunctions that result from various types of excesses and deficiencies:

Organ	Excess	Dysfunction
Liver	Excessive drinking, drug use, anger	Burning and hardening of liver, uncontrollable tremors
Heart	Too many thrills, excitement, mental stress	Heart attack, arrhythmia, emotional depletion
Spleen	Excessive stress, worry, and thinking	Chronic digestive problems, inability to absorb nutrients, lack of decisive action, inability to make decisions
Lungs	Excessive grief and sadness, or withholding grief	Immune deficiency, asthma, other respiratory problems

Organ	Excess	Dysfunction
Kidneys	Extreme or chronic fear and anxiety, excessive sexual intercourse	Premature aging, impotence, early menopause, reproductive problems

Any disruption of the intrinsic pathway of the qi stream will gradually deplete the body of its nutrients, leading to decline and degeneration.

Once, my teacher was asked by a patient, "Doctor, what is the perfect diet?"

"Not very much," he answered. In other words, do not eat any type of food to excess. It is unhealthy to eat too much bread, sugar, or meat. Similarly, rather than stuffing in a large meal at one sitting, it is healthier to eat smaller meals. How wonderful, the secret to healthy eating is expressed by these three words: Not very much.

Organ	Deficiencies	Dysfunctions
Liver	Chronic liver infections, fatigue from extreme physical labor, lack of sexual hormones	Insomnia, recurring nightmares, ringing in the ears, numbness in the extremities, menopausal symptoms
Heart	Blocked or deficient blood flow to heart, deep psychological trauma— as in victims of childhood and sexual abuse	Chest pain, tongue turn purplish, bruised nails, coldness in fingers and toes, panic attacks, mental disorders, low self-esteem
Spleen	Malnourishment, heavy blood loss due to abnormal menstruation, surgery, or internal hemorrhaging	Weak voice, inability to heal or recover from sickness. Weakness in muscular strength, and loose, watery stools

Organ	Deficiencies	Dysfunctions
Lungs	Chronic lung infections, inhaling toxic fumes, smoking, long-term exposure to cold and wet conditions	Fluid in the lungs, shortness of breath, dry cough, edema, inability to organize daily activities
Kidneys	Chronic mental, physical, or environmental stresses, chronic urinary tract or kidney infections, premature birth, neonatal malnourishment	Chronic fatigue, loose teeth, bleeding gums, lower back and/or knee pain, frequent urination, night sweats, hair falling out, morning diarrhea

The therapeutic principle of Healing Sounds Qigong is to bring the organs from their excessive or deficient state back to homeostasis. This approach is parallel to repairing a broken thermostat. In this case, one's house will either become too hot or too cold. By practicing the healing sounds, we reawaken our internal sensors and feedback system, thus returning the organs to their natural state of balance and health.[1]

Rejuvenation and Regeneration

For the Taoist, healing is fundamentally a regenerative process, with the goal of returning the organs and qi to their original state of free flow and harmony. Once the internal balance and homeostasis between the organs is established, health is regained.

The Taoist Six Healing Sounds are one method of restoring the organs and qi flow to their original pristine state. This is achieved through the following components of the Six Healing Sounds Qigong process:

- Meditation for each organ
- Individual organic sound to resonate with the organ
- Movement to enhance the freedom of breath and blood flow

These three components are like three strands of colorful thread. By interweaving them in the unique practice of the Six Healing Sounds Qigong, we can recuperate and rejuvenate our life force and even grow younger like the legendary alchemist Merlin.[2]

Alchemical Ritual: Taoist Principles of Health and Therapeutics

"I am a simple woman. I can't deal with all this academic, intellectual learning!" one of my students said to me.

"Then just make a cup of cocoa," I told her.

The Taoist principles of body function are as simple as making a cup of good hot chocolate. If you know how to do that, then you know the foundation of healing. In order to understand the relationship of the body's inner functions, we create a paradigm of our inner body with its internal organs. And we illustrate it as a dynamic process that we call the alchemical ritual of making a cup of hot cocoa, my favorite drink.

Alchemy is nothing other than transmuting your inner life force so that it tastes good. Taste your own life force, and I bet that some of you will find that your life tastes too hot, too spicy, or too salty. Or sometimes, we have too many condiments and not enough basic stock—too many good gestures and not enough real compassionate response—but we do not notice that we are missing something.

I once taught a student how to make some good old-fashioned chicken broth for her cold. I said to her, "Take half a pound of chicken cutlet, half a ginger root, and half a scallion, put it in a pot, and boil it for twenty minutes." That evening, I got a call from her.

She said, "What happened to your recipe? I put all the ingredients in the pot and heated it for twenty minutes, but there's no liquid for soup. I don't know what I did wrong."

I said, "Well, I told you to put in chicken, ginger, and scallion; how much water did you add?"

And she asked, "What water?"

She had neglected to add water to the pot. Without water, there is no chicken broth. I had assumed that she would know this basic fact, so I didn't bother to include water in the recipe. Similarly, one might be blind to a simple, obvious ingredient that is missing from one's life, even though it might be very evident to others. Attentive awareness in daily actions is a common missing ingredient in life. To be aware is as essential as having water in making chicken broth.

To make a cup of hot cocoa with awareness, you must know the alchemical ritual's inner geography, as is shown in the illustration below.

MAKING A CUP OF HOT COCOA

In this alchemical rite of cocoa, we create a visual representation of our organs. The different vessels are our internal organs, and the fluid that is being circulated is our life force and essence, our qi. This life force, qi, is circulated between the different organs—pouring from one organ into another to achieve transformation and enrichment of the qi, so the body can absorb it.

Water is poured from the wooden bowl, the liver, to be heated by the heart fire. This energized water then has the ability to dissolve the granular cocoa, so the spleen can store the nutrients. Through the gentle swirling of the water, the cocoa powder is dissolved in the next container, the milky silver bowl of the lungs.

The milk added to the cocoa gives it its rich flavor and coolness. After that, it is poured into the black teapot of the kidney to be distributed into three little cups. The three little cups represent the triple heater—upper, lower, and middle.

In this alchemical ritual, if any part is missing, it will create a not very tasty hot cocoa. This is parallel to a state of mild disharmony; in TCM, disharmony is equated with sickness.

For example, if the heart's fire is not strong enough to heat the water from the liver, then the cocoa won't dissolve and you will get lumpy hot cocoa. This lumpiness will result in a general sense of congestion. In order to have fluid, open energy, the heart's fire needs to be free and burning brightly. Then you get good, hot, smooth cocoa and a sense of joyousness that emanates outward.

How does the wooden bowl represent the liver? The liver has the quality of growth and connectivity, like wood. The candle with the flame is the heart, the fire. The yellow bowl is the spleen that stores the goodies that it likes to eat, the sweet cocoa powder. The silver bowl is the lung. It stores the cool, rich liquid of milk. Some of us have too much of that, and we cough it up as mucus—it's white. And when it is fermented like yogurt, it becomes yellow: bronchitis.

The fifth vessel is the kidney, represented by a black iron teapot. The teapot is totally enclosed, with only a spout for pouring out. This enables the distribution of the fluid into the last vessel, the three cups that represent the triple heater, one for each part of the body (upper, middle, and lower).

Each Healing Sound corresponds to an individual organ and will be explained in detail in the following chapters.

The chart below summarizes the organs' elements and characteristics.

Organ/Sound	Element	Function
Liver/XU	Wood	Connectivity
Heart/HO	Fire	Warming, consciousness
Spleen/FU	Earth	Storage
Lungs/XI	Metal	Cooling
Kidney/CHU	Water	Distribution
Triple heater/HEY	Chimera fire	Lymphatic circulation

ALCHEMICAL MEDITATION:

MAKING A CUP OF INNER COCOA

Health requires that your internal energy pass from one vessel to another without any blockage, without any excess, and without any disruption of the movement of the organs. The following is a meditation on the alchemical ritual of making hot cocoa.

This alchemical visualization process can be done almost anywhere—on a train or plane or even before the start of a movie—as long as it is a safe place. It is possible to nourish our internal organs with this simple visualization of making a cup of cocoa.

With your eyes closed, inhale and exhale. Take a moment and relax, letting go of any inner tension. Let your hands rest in your lap. Now imagine that in your right hand you are holding a wooden bowl—this symbolizes your liver. Slowly raise your right hand to the level of your solar plexus. You are holding a bowl filled with cool, pristine spring water. Slowly turn your right hand and pour the cool water from the bowl into the heart. Visualize the heart as a red vessel with a small golden flame heating it from underneath. The golden flame represents the heart's warming function. Take a few breaths. Feel a wonderful sense of joy and warmth radiating from your heart as the water within is being warmed up. Now, lower your right hand, with the palm facing down, to the left side of your rib cage at the stomach/spleen area. Visualize that the warm heart's water is gently emptied into the yellow bowl of the spleen, which already holds the sweet cocoa powder. Now tenderly rub your stomach with your right palm as if you were mixing the ingredients thoroughly. Take a moment and just imagine the sweetness of the cocoa nourishing your spleen and stomach. Inhale and feel how the refreshing breaths from the lungs suffuse the spleen like cool milk enriching the cocoa. Now, return your right hand to your lap, palm up. Visualize the cocoa flowing down into the black teapot of the kidneys. A sense of peace and tranquillity settles within you, like an early morning summer mist. Finally, visualize the cocoa dispersing into the three regions: navel, diaphragm, and upper chest. As your raise your hands with the palms together to these three regions, at each level, silently offer the cocoa to all sentient beings. Now, take a drink of the inner cocoa that you made. How does it taste?

Healing Story: Baptism at White Cloud Mountain

"Why don't you both stay here, and we can all share the bed to-gether," suggested my mother as she pointed to a twin-size bed in our old house in China. "That would save you money on a hotel."

As I translated the words to my wife, Janet, her eyes widened in horror. Being of European descent, she was not accustomed to Chinese culture, particularly our family's frugality.

"There is no way that we can all fit in that bed." She spoke softly to me from the side of her mouth.

"We would not dream of being such an inconvenience to you, Mom. It is better if we stay in a hotel." I declined my mother's offer.

After Janet and I got married, I wanted to take her back to China to visit my old home and pay homage to some of my relatives. Since I had immigrated to the United States as young boy, I had not been back for more then twenty years. Of course, news of such a trip was hard to keep secret. My mother got wind of it and offered to join us and help us meet with our relatives back in China.

After twenty hours of traveling by plane and train, and dodging having to share a bed with my mother, Janet and I finally collapsed in our air-conditioned room at the China Hotel. We were finally alone. As I watched Janet lying asleep next to me, I suddenly realized what my mother had been trying to do: train Janet to be a frugal Chinese wife.

One time, my mother related to me something my grandmother had told her: "In the old days, a wife was never given a full meal until she reached the age of fifty. She would serve the meal to her family first and then eat the leftovers afterward." Amid disquieting images of emaciated women, I drifted off to sleep.

Early the next morning, my mother arrived with our laundry—she had washed all the clothes by hand. I was sure that was another lesson in frugality. After breakfast, we decided that we would all go sightseeing. Our first stop would be White Cloud Mountain just outside the city.

August in Guangzhou, where the temperature averaged 100 degrees, was dangerous. Under the hot sun, with humidity so thick it felt as if we were being smothered by a wet handkerchief, we climbed the tortuous mountain path. Halfway up, we had finished every drop of water from our canteen. I noticed that Janet's face was flushed and that she was evidently suffering from great thirst.

"Remember the time we walked along Delancey Street, with vendors displaying barrels of pickles right on the sidewalk? We had the best pickle there," I said, trying to distract her from her thirst.

"Yes, it was a hot day, but not as hot as now. That pickle tasted like a little burst of sunshine. It was both sweet and sour at the same time," Janet replied, starting to salivate.

"After World War II, your father and I used to carry water to sell along this very path. We would get up at three A.M. and walk three miles with a big bucket of water halfway up the mountain. It was very good business but hard work." My mother seemed impervious to thirst or fatigue. "Now there are no water sellers around. People nowadays are just too lazy to earn an honest living," she added.

Trying to slake Janet's thirst, I kept steering our conversation to food in order to get her to salivate, or at least to keep her parched throat in abeyance till we arrived at the top of the mountain. Fortunately, I had read an old story about how a Chinese general had kept his troops from dying of thirst. He kept promising the soldiers that not very far ahead of them there was a grove of plum trees laden with juicy plums. As the soldiers fantasized about the plums, they started to salivate. Their own saliva helped to slake their thirst until finally they reached a mountain stream.

I had almost run out of stories of sour pickles, coleslaw, and such when, just in time, we reached the plateau of White Cloud Mountain. Lo and behold, nestled beneath an old banyan tree was a moss-green cobblestone well, the Nine-Dragon Well. It is rare to find such a well on top of a mountain. According to legend, a powerful alchemist had conjured the well out of the hard ground of the mountain. The water of the Nine-Dragon Well is renowned far and wide as the best mineral water, with wonderful curative powers. This was the only water that we drank in China without boiling first. Miraculously, we did not get sick.

After paying the well attendant, we were given a red plastic bucket. As I lowered it into the well, suddenly three obsidian-black carps with golden eyes loomed up. They were suspended in utter stillness and seemed to be fixed in space and time, like some ancient spirits conjured up with the Nine-Dragon Well a thousand years ago. I muttered my gratitude to these guardians of the well as I gingerly hoisted a brimming bucket of liquid light.

"Ah, that is the best water I've ever tasted in my life!" Janet cried. After gulping down nearly a quart of water, she became almost euphoric. All her fatigue and the stress of traveling with her mother-in-law seemed to evaporate.

As the cool, pristine watery mountain essence filled me, I felt every cell in my body tingle as if a mild electricity had run through it, permeating each cell with a soft white light, rendering it translucent like shimmering leaves with sunlight shining through.

Meanwhile, my mother had dipped a towel in the remaining water and nonchalantly started to give herself a sponge bath, right there in public. Furtively, I glanced around, and it seemed that almost everyone was also cleansing themselves in the same way. Joining in this communal rite of baptism, I felt as though I had been transported to some magical mountaintop, with silken clouds so close that I could almost brush them with my fingers. In an instant, I was transformed from a tourist into a pilgrim, and this journey became a pilgrimage, an homage to my own ancestral spirits.

Afterward, we filled a small vial of the Nine-Dragon Well water and brought it back home.

Now, on hot, sultry summer days I'll spice up my tea with just a drop or two of this ambrosia. Once more, I can almost taste the spark of electricity on my tongue, and an immeasurable longing for the earth's ancient magic wells up within me.

3
PRINCIPLES OF CORE
HARMONICS

Imagine a lavender droplet
Immersed in water, diffusing.
It branches into infinitesimal tendrils,
Permeating the body of water.

Imagine at the core of our being
Emitting a single sound, "ah,"
That rings the earth's spheric sky like a bell.
Its basso reverberation engulfs dark space and stars.

Imagine a simple wave of the hand
Fired up by a thousand tendrils of nerves,
Sending ripples from fingers to toes.

S O F A R , no one has been able to completely map out the laws of the living body in motion. For a living body possesses an inner universe wholly indescribable by Newtonian physics. Scientists call the study of the living body in motion kinesiology. I remember from my student days how clinical and cold those academic textbooks were, describing how "the supination of the metatarsal arch causes the prolapse of the foot." How can you deconstruct the grace of Nijinsky's *grand jeté* to just bones and ligaments?

Physical and Inner Pairings

In qigong movement, six pairs of synergetic components align with each other. These pairings are similar to the striking of two notes on a piano to create a harmonic chord. The physical pairings are:

- Shoulders and hips
- Elbows and knees
- Feet and hands

The inner pairings are:

- Breath and physical movement
- Intention and eyes
- Numen and sexual essence[1]

SHOULDERS AND HIPS

When doing Qigong in a standing or seated position, it is important to line up the shoulders with the hips. Imagine that you are stacking a column of books. The shoulders should be stacked directly above the hips (see figs. 3.1 and 3.2).

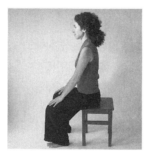 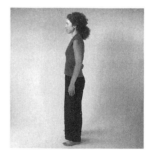

FIGURE 3.1   FIGURE 3.2

ELBOWS AND KNEES

When doing Qigong movements, keep the elbows in alignment with the knees. Imagine that there is an invisible line attached between them. For example, imagine a puppet with its elbow joints linked to its knee joints by a wire. When the elbow moves, the knee moves at the same time.

FEET AND HANDS

In Qigong, it's important to keep the hands in the same plane of action as the feet. For example, imagine taking a simple stretch like a big yawn. As you stretch your hands above your head, the hands should not reach behind the plane of your feet. Many unnecessary lower back strains result from overreaching of the hands behind the plane of the feet.

These three sets of physical pairings—the shoulders and hips, elbows and knees, and hands and feet—serve as basic guidelines in Qigong practice. Being aware of how these three physical pairs interact with each other during every exercise will help prevent overstraining and injury.

BREATH AND MOVEMENT

Qigong means "breath work." In other words, as you move, you must also breathe in synchrony with the movement. This may seem simplistic, but I have frequently observed that my beginning students tend to hold their breath. A simple self-diagnosis is to notice how often you hold your breath throughout the day. In general, when doing Qigong, inhale as you stretch your arms away from the body. Exhale as you gather your arms, as if hugging yourself. Inhale as your body rises up. Exhale as you lower the body.

These general guidelines serve as useful signposts for beginners practicing the Healing Sounds movements. There will be exceptions. During practice, simply place your awareness on your breathing while moving. Breathing is a spontaneous natural function. If you are aware of your respiration, this very awareness will free up tension in your body. Once old habitual blockages—holding the stomach in or pulling the shoulders back—are released, natural spontaneous breathing will be integrated with your movements.

INTENTION AND EYES

Imagine that you are shooting a basketball. You must aim your shot before you throw the ball. This is done by looking first at your target, the basket. During physical movement, look but don't stare at your fingertips; such seeing helps to transmit the mental intention of movement to your hands. Here is a simple exercise: wave your hand as if greeting someone. Now, repeat the action. While lifting your hand, let your eyes follow your fingertips. Compare the difference between the two gestures. You will find in the second gesture a keener sense of self-awareness. When we keep the hands in our line of vision, qi energy is directed to the fingertips; this helps to open our internal energetic pathways. This opening of our energetic pathways is the principle of healing in the science of acupuncture. We can accomplish similar results just by keeping our hands in our line of vision! Unbelievable, but true.

NUMEN AND SEXUAL ESSENCE

Numen is the spiritual aspect of ourselves. Sexual essence is the physical life force, the foundation of our existence. In Taoist alchemy, this last pairing between numen and sexual essence is represented by the Ouroboros,[2] the serpent that devours its own tail. It is an alchemical regenerative cycle that transmutes the coarse sexual essence from its physical state to a higher spiritual state of numinous function. This is represented by the alchemical process of transmuting lead into gold, body into mind, and mortality into immortality. Here lies the magnum opus of all Taoist cultivations.

Envision these six pairings as six tacks holding and stretching smooth the fabric of a canvas. We can use the six synergetic pairs to verify and assess our posture and state of mind. Similarly, by keeping these six pairings in our consciousness, we create a smooth state of awareness during movement. When there is total harmony between the six pairs, we have a palpable sense of what is normally imperceptible, a glacial flow of sensation spreading out into space. Suddenly, the mover who moved dissolves. Subject and object, mind and body dissolve; there is just this one moment, suspended beyond time and space.

Eight Breath Integrals

The eight breath integrals are the eight most important body regions associated with breathing freely. In order to practice the Taoist Healing Sounds properly, one must pay attention to the eight breath integrals and keep them in a state of relaxation. This is comparable to properly tuning the strings of a cello before you can perform great music. The following process tunes the eight integral "strings" for proper breathing:

1. *Respiratory diaphragm.* The diaphragm is like a rubber band. During inhalation it stretches taut, and when we exhale it releases. As it releases, the diaphragm floats way up under the ribs and up to the bottom of the heart, giving the liver room to expand during exhalation. An important aspect of a full breath is that it allows the diaphragm to massage our internal organs. Place your hands on your abdomen and take a deep breath in and out. Observe how your hands move up and down as you breathe. The respiratory diaphragm contracting and releasing accomplishes that action.

2. *Lungs.* The lungs have the largest surface area of any internal organ. Imagine that they are like a wet sponge filled with fluid and air (the common notion that the lungs resemble balloons is misleading). Healthy lungs must be able to expel as much fluid and gas as possible, to allow fresh air to come in. Therefore, the principle of good breathing relies on a thorough exhalation, while the inhalation will come naturally and spontaneously without too much force.

3. *Ribs.* The ribs surround the lungs like the frame of a canoe. As they should be free to expand, the muscles between them must be soft

and not tight. The shoulders have to be relaxed and lowered to allow the free-floating action of the ribs during respiration and the practice of the Healing Sounds.

4. *Bronchi.* Place your palms just underneath your throat, on the top of your sternum, with your fingers pointing down. Now spread your fingers and imagine that your fingers are tubes that extend down through your lungs. This mimics the pathway of the bronchi, which are two branching tubes that connect with each lung.

5. *Throat and larynx.* The larynx is the voice box. It is like a tollbooth, allowing the air to enter and exit. As the air exits, it creates a vibration, which becomes sound and speech. There is an unconscious habit of shutting the larynx and tensing the throat when one is silent. Keep them open at all times, especially during inhalation.

6. *Soft palate.* The soft palate is located at the back of the roof of your mouth. It is one component in shaping and giving resonance to speech and singing, and it is important to keep it soft and round while doing the Healing Sounds.

7. *Tongue.* The tongue actually extends to the back of the throat. It is very important to keep the tongue soft and relaxed when doing the Healing Sounds.

8. *Jaw and lips.* Allow the jaw to droop as if you are drunk. Keep the lips soft, as if you are being kissed.

These eight breath integrals are very important for freeing your breath. Go through them silently as you inhale and exhale. Feel how the diaphragm goes up and down, how the ribs expand and contract, how the lungs and bronchi soften, the throat and larynx relax, the soft palate and tongue release, and the jaw and lips let go. Think of the eight breath integrals as musicians playing in an orchestra. Feel how they synchronize and move with each other as you do the Healing Sounds. This is an indication that they are in a state of dynamic harmony.

These are the fundamentals of breathing when practicing the Healing Sounds. They should be done with natural ease and without artificial or habitual tensions. In the movie *Meetings with Remarkable*

Men (1979), a Sufi master advised G. I. Gurdjieff that he should abandon all his artificial breathing exercises and training because this way of breathing was forced and unnatural and could cause him great harm. Many teachers of breathing mislead others due to their own lack of understanding of the breathing mechanism. Gurdjieff related this story as a warning to the ignorant practitioners of traditional breathing exercises.

Finally, the skillful use of sound during breathing will give the student a clear sense of good healthy breath. After all, when you sing out the AH sound, you are really breathing out. And if this AH sound has a crystal bell-like resonance, then it verifies that you have indeed exhaled correctly without tension. On the other hand, if the AH sound has a muffled, choked thickness, as if you were singing under a blanket, this signifies too much tension during the exhalation. In this way, the Six Healing Sounds provide us with a safe, effective, and clear way to do breathing practice.

Guide to the Six Healing Sounds Practice

Traveling on a mountain path,
I met a man who was building a great pile of wood.
"What, may I ask, are you trying to do?"
"Oh, I am making a great fire," he replied with a self-satisfied smile.
"How long have you been gathering wood?"
"All my life!"
"When will you light the fire?" I asked.
"I am too busy gathering wood. And what do you mean by lighting a
  fire?" His eyes opened wide with confusion.
Shaking my head, I walked on as the man placed another load of
  wood on his growing pile.

Gathering the dry wood of book knowledge will not cause the fire of wisdom to ignite. Only when you take the written words and put them into practice do they combust and come alive. The Tao of learning does not involve fixating on achieving certain specific goals. Learning is more like taking an after-dinner stroll along a riverbank. Let your feet guide you where they will without guilty thoughts about not doing it right.

The overall aim of Qigong healing is to strengthen and awaken your body's own immune and spontaneous healing systems, so that they can deal with the sickness at hand to realize a full rejuvenation of aliveness.

TIME OF PRACTICE

After you have read a few chapters, it is important that you actually get up and try some of the movements. By experiencing the Qigong exercises, you will retain and feel the benefits directly in your body.

Establish a daily practice; this is crucial. As with much of Taoist Qigong, there are optimal times at which to engage in the practice in order to enhance the overall effect. In general, the best times to practice the Healing Sounds are between 11:00 P.M. and 1:00 A.M., and between 4:30 A.M. and 5:30 A.M. At these times, all the body systems are cleared of environmental disturbances. Of course, those times originated in an ancient agrarian society. For us today, early morning is a good time. Practicing before you go to work creates a gentle routine of waking up slowly. You will find that if you establish a simple morning routine of Healing Sounds practice, you will have more energy throughout the day to deal with the daily stress of work. If it is not possible to practice then, pick a regular period of free time. Qigong practice is like boiling water in order to purify it: it needs to be done for at least twenty minutes in order for the health benefits to occur. Poor times to practice are immediately before or after eating, before or after sexual intercourse, after drinking alcohol, or in a state of heightened emotion, for instance, when angered.

POSTURE

Maintaining proper posture during practice is very important. The goal of the postures is to maintain a sense of release and opening of all the joints in your body. Any posture that requires unnatural or habitual muscular tension—for example, sucking in your belly to make it look flat or tucking in the tailbone—usually wastes energy and causes more harm than benefit. In some instances, the muscular tension will block your natural way of breathing. However, do not simply allow the body to collapse. Even though it may feel comfortable, this is merely letting the body fall into its old habitual patterns.

There are three major postures you can assume in the practice of the Healing Sounds: standing, seated, and supine positions.

Standing

Imagine that you are standing on the center of a seesaw with your feet approximately shoulder width apart. Make sure your weight is distributed equally between your feet. Then, visualize that a small balloon is tied to your head, gently lifting it. This small balloon frees your neck of all tension, and you begin to feel lightness in your whole body (see fig. 3.3).

Experiment with standing and with releasing all unnatural tension. Always keep your eyes slightly open. Do not stand in any place that is dangerous, such as near an open window, and make sure that there are no sharp objects behind or in front of you, in case you fall.

Sitting

The Healing Sounds can also be done in a sitting position. You should sit on the edge of your chair with your feet flat on the floor. Begin with your hands on your knees. Visualize the balloon attached to your head as described in the standing posture (see fig. 3.4).

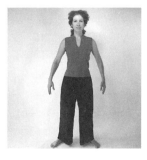
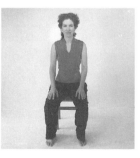

FIGURE 3.3   FIGURE 3.4

Supine

In China, patients are taught Healing Sounds Qigong while they are lying in bed. Lie on a soft, firm rug or yoga mat. Prop up your head with a small pillow or cushion so that it is not tilted back. Bend your knees and place your feet flat on the mat. Make sure there is a fist-width space between your knees. This open space will help to create a flow of energy from the pelvis to the feet. Sense your shoulders sinking into the ground. Now use the balloon visualization as described in the standing posture, stretching the neck to elongate the spine.

Preparatory Practices

Four preparatory practices for the Healing Sounds are presented in this section: the Gatha of Awareness, the Golden Light Meditation, the Himalayan AH sound, and the Six Sounds Gatha. They serve as preliminary templates for the Healing Sounds practices in the later chapters.

GATHA OF AWARENESS

This gatha may be recited before the practice of any of the Healing Sounds. It serves as a way of channeling your mind to prepare you for the journey of healing.

> Let body return to body,
> Let mind return to mind,
> Let being return to being,
> Let breath return to breath,
> Let all things return to themselves.
>
> All effort comes to an end.
> Awareness emerges like blue sky.
>
> Being aware has no self.
> Being aware has no beginning.

Being aware has no time.
In a single moment of awareness,
    the whole universe is awakened.

You may repeat the gatha up to three times. When you have finished, you may proceed to the Golden Light Meditation.

GOLDEN LIGHT MEDITATION

Sit at ease. Inhale deeply, and then exhale as much as you can. Get rid of all of the exhaust. Again, inhale . . . and exhale. Blow out your breath. Inhale. Exhale.

Now gently lengthen your spine, letting your eyes close. Allow the tip of your tongue to touch your palate. If you have any heart problems or high blood pressure, lower the tip of the tongue to touch the bottom of your mouth.

Take a deep breath, as if smelling the sweet after-fragrance of a drizzling autumn rain. As you inhale, imagine your head opening up like a flower. The top of your head is open and the drizzling rain becomes a golden stream entering your brain. Allow the golden fluid to fill and illuminate your brain, and then allow the fluid to drip down through the brain stem to the tip of your tongue and down to the root of your tongue into your throat, letting it drop down into your heart. As soon as you feel the golden stream enter your heart, inhale and allow the heart to gently contract and then expand. As the heart opens like a flower, a light, joyous feeling emanates to the rest of your body. Let this joy overflow your heart and pour down gently into your abdomen.

The golden fluid has been warmed by the heart, so now your belly starts to grow warm, as if a gentle morning light is shining on it. The same warmth penetrates from the front of your abdomen to your lower back, soothing your lower back. Now let this sense of warmth move down the inside of your legs; relax the thighs as the sensation of warmth trickles down; as if a golden fluid is flowing down the insides of your legs. Now, allow the knees to relax, then the calves, and finally all the way down to the bottom of your feet.

Now, imagine a golden stream filling from the top of your head to the soles of the feet and your whole body shimmering with a brilliant light. Allow this amber light to emanate from within you, embracing and permeating every cell of your body. Merge with the light, then allow spontaneous healing to occur.

HIMALAYAN *AH* SOUND

Freeing one's voice comes from freeing one's breath. The basic principle of the Healing Sounds is freeing the breath. By using the sound as a feedback, we are able to learn the quality and characteristic of our breathing. One way of doing this is through the use of the Himalayan AH sound.

Remain in the state of deep relaxation you reached by doing the Golden Light Meditation, and stay as comfortable as possible. Imagine that after a month's hard journey, you have finally arrived at the top of Mount Everest, and, standing there at the peak, you see the panorama of the Himalayas. Your mouth drops open and the breathy sound of AH is released from you. Now breathing in, maintain the shape of the mouth, as if you were inhaling with the AH sound. You look at the panorama and your mouth just drops open and you say AH.

Now repeat that, this time with your eyes rolling slightly up. Let your jaw drop and your throat open. As you inhale, be sure that you do not suck in your breath. Imagine that you are like an empty vase submerged in a pool of cool water and that the air just pours effortlessly into your lungs. Look up slightly, inhale, and say AH.

Now you may want to gently tap your chest with your fingers, like a pianist touching the keys or like a good antiques buyer checking out the quality of the wood. Tap it gently on both sides to free up any constriction. At a certain moment, you will feel a sudden release in tension.

Repeat the AH again. Visualize your diaphragm as a big rubber band, and, as you inhale, stretch that imaginary rubber band downward. Then, as you exhale, imagine that the rubber band releases and shoots upward and the breath escapes. At the end of the exhalation, the diaphragm is at ease and there is a slight pulse of three heartbeats when the whole body is at rest. It is as if there is a twilight zone between inhaling and exhaling. Let that pause last.

Repeat once more. This time inhale with the same AH sound in your mind, and then exhale with the AH sound as before.

Now you may begin to feel a slight dizziness. If it is not excessive and if you do not feel too much discomfort, that is a natural sign of your brain being oxygenated. In a moment, this giddiness will pass. If not, sit or lie down till it passes.

You may practice the AH sound a few more times. When you have done this sufficiently and feel comfortable, you may proceed to the next section, the practice of the Six Healing Sounds themselves.

SIX SOUNDS GATHA

Be aware of the eight breath integrals. Let them function like eight horses working in synergy, in cooperation. Do not squeeze your ribs while inhaling; let the ribs float freely, relaxed. Do not tense your throat when you are exhaling; let it stay open. Keep these things in mind. These are the fundamentals of freeing the breath and breathing naturally. They serve as the foundation of our Healing Sounds practice. The Healing Sounds are not magical incantations. If you do them incorrectly, breathing poorly, you will not derive any health benefit from them, so it is important to do the practice with full, free breath.

We will now experiment with the Six Healing Sounds. They are as follows:

- The first sound is for the liver, the sound XU.
- The second sound is for the heart, the sound HO.
- The third sound is for the spleen, the sound FU.
- The fourth sound is for the lungs, the sound XI.
- The fifth sound is for the kidneys, the sound CHU.
- The sixth sound is for the triple heater, the sound HEY.

Try each sound individually a few times. Then, to practice the sounds together, you may recite the Six Sounds Gatha:

> xu to hush the liver
> ho to open the heart
> fu to cool the spleen
> xi to tease the lungs
> chu to release the kidneys
> hey to wake up the triple heater
>
>
> xu, ho, fu, xi, chu, hey
> xu, ho, fu, xi, chu, hey
> xu, ho, fu, xi, chu, hey

General Guidelines for Healing Sounds Meditation

Before practicing the Healing Sounds for each organ as described in the next chapters, follow these general guidelines as a preparation:

- Find a low stool or a chair so that your feet can rest firmly on the floor. For meditation or the relaxation process, never sit for long periods with your feet dangling in the air. This will cause the blood to drain to the feet, and with no pressure from the floor it is very difficult for the venous blood to return to the heart.
- Spread your knees to the width of your shoulders.
- Rest your hands on your knees with palms down. Or you can rest your hands on your thighs with the palms up if you find this more comfortable.
- Move your pelvis so that you are sitting on the edge of the seat. (Men should make sure their testicles hang freely and are not pressed against the chair.) If you let your back rest against the chair back, this will cause the lumbar spine to collapse and block the flow of qi along the spinal column. This way of sitting on the edge (the Taoists call it "precarious sitting") demands that we pay

attention to our alignment in the seated posture. You will notice how, in the lower back, the lumbar vertebrae become free and undulate with each breath. This precarious sitting can also be done on a meditation cushion.

- Let your spine be naturally erect, like an unstrung bow. Let all the vertebrae be strung loosely, hanging freely like a strand of pearls. When standing or sitting, rotate the trunk of the body in a circular motion. This will help to free and warm up the lumbar vertebrae of the lower back.

- Drop the ribs as you exhale, as if you are folding in the ribs of an umbrella. Use your palms and gently tap the ribs to release tension of the intercostal muscles between the ribs. Gently run your right palm over your stomach area to warm up the spleen and help its energy to flow.

- Soften your heart and chest. The chest should not be puffed up, nor should it be collapsed.

- Tap your fingers gently against your sternum. This will help release any tension in the region. Sometimes excessive tension in the chest will cause the heartbeat to quicken. Softening the heart will reduce the heart rate.

- Relax the back of your neck by imagining that your head is like a buoy floating on the water. Tuck your chin in very slightly to help relax the neck further.

- Touch the tip of your tongue to the roof of your mouth, the upper palate. (Variations: If you have a heart problem, touch the tongue to the bottom palate. If you would like to lose weight, let the tongue hang freely in the middle of the mouth without touching the palate.)

- Lower your eyelids, but keep them open a tiny crack, so that you can see a forty-five-degree angle down in front of you. The Taoist masters called this area "where the cow lies down." (A cow will not lie down any closer to you than that distance away.) Do not close your eyes completely—this will cause your mind to wander. This also helps to entice the qi down the body from the head, and centers the mind on the body.

Healing Sound Story: California Dreaming

At the end of a Healing Sounds workshop I conducted in California, one of the participants, Crystal, approached me. Her eyes were shiny and filled with excitement.

"Master Hon, I want you to know that many lifetimes ago, we knew each other. I was your Taoist teacher," she confided in me, while other students stood around us in stony silence.

"Oh, I am so glad that we have met again, my teacher. I hope that I can repay your kindness by reminding you of what you have forgotten," I replied without missing a beat and folded my palms together in gratitude at having met my old master again after so many lifetimes.

Later on, Crystal volunteered to be my personal assistant and chauffeur. As we were driving down a busy avenue, we passed through a series of intersections. At the third one, Crystal drove through a red light, and I must have involuntarily grasped my seat belt. Noting my concern, Crystal said with a slight chuckle, "Oh well, two out of three ain't bad."

I suddenly realized that for her, an evolved being who could remember her many past lives, it would be acceptable if we were struck by a car. After all, there are still many more lives to live. From then on, although Crystal became one of my most faithful and caring assistants, she would never drive me again.

I have often wondered whether the Healing Sounds had evoked or provoked Crystal's past-life recollection. If so, this would be an extraordinary property of the Healing Sounds that I hadn't anticipated.

PRELUDE TO THE HEALING SOUNDS: CARVING AN OX

WHEN THE PRINCE OF WEI decided to research the art of nourishing life, he needed to look no further than his kitchen.

"I would like to hear the art of life. What is the best way to nourish life?" asked the Prince.

The chef lovingly held his knife up to show the prince.

"The blade looks brand new!"

"Your lordship, I have been using this blade for thirty years, and it hasn't been sharpened since the very first day!

"In the beginning, when I started working as an apprentice, I saw only the ox carcass. I would slice into the bones and tendons, and in a few days my blade would be dull. The frequent sharpening of the blade caused me to replace my knife every six months. Then I embarked on my study of the ox. For three years, I analyzed the structures hidden beneath the skin, where the bones meet and the sinews connect. I was so focused that I would no longer see a whole ox but only its interrelated parts. I trained myself to guide the blade to slice through the space between the joints and tendons. Since my blade sailed through the emptiness between sinews and bone without meeting any resistance, its sharpness was never dulled. So it never needed sharpening.

"Now, when I encounter difficult knotted structures, emptying my mind, I let my hands guide me to the small cavities and crevices. Then everything drops away naturally like mulberry leaves falling in autumn rain. As the tangled mess dissolves, I stand still in the radiant presence of the void." With these last words, the old chef bowed and departed.

"Ah, how simple it is indeed. To shrink our ego to the fine edge of a blade and seek out the emptiness that exists in all situations. Thus we do not flounder and squander our life force pitting it against the hard rock of ambition."

When a complex situation is resolved by a complicated solution, often the solution will generate secondary complications. Sometimes a simple primordial sound uttered with perfection can ignite our spontaneous healing response.

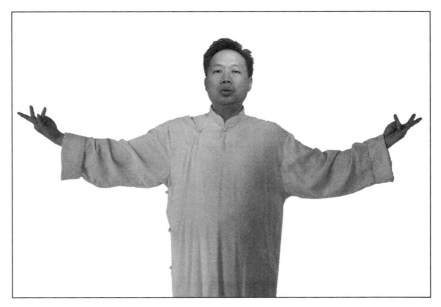

Liver

4

LIVER: THE TREE OF LIFE

Sitting by the river in springtime,
Gurgling sound of glacial water,
A breath from heaven
Soothes the thousand little fires within.

IN TAOIST PRACTICE, there is no distinction between the profound and the mundane. The deepest truth is available in the simplest action, such as in preparing a cup of hot cocoa. To know that the profoundest truth starts with ordinary activity is the heart of awakened living.

In the alchemical ritual, we create a paradigm of the six organs of our inner body. This gives us an overview of the Chinese principles of the organs' functions. The different vessels and containers represent the different organs; and the fluids, represented by the water, are circulated between the organs, pouring from one to the other, transforming them, nourishing them, and creating the final product that our body can absorb and be nourished by.

Through the alchemical ritual of making a cup of hot cocoa, we can begin to understand the function of the liver. First, we use a wooden bowl in order to store the water, because the first function of the liver is storage and adjustment or detoxification of blood in the body. When you are at rest, most of the blood returns to the liver. When you arise, you open your eyes, and the liver pumps out the blood that is stored in the organ to the heart. So any sickness that is blood related will have an effect on the liver. For example, in TCM, hepatitis is fundamentally a liver problem due to a poisoning of the blood. Another blood syndrome is dysfunction of the menstrual cycle. When a woman has too much or too little menstrual flow, it is because the liver is not functioning properly.

Second, we use the wooden bowl because of the wood-element characteristic of the liver. What characteristics does wood have? On the one hand, wood is strong and binding, like a vine. But wood also has the characteristic of movement. Indeed, of all the five elements, wood is the most mobile besides water. So the liver controls not only the binding agents of our physical body (such as the fascia and ligaments) but also the structures that enable movement (such as muscles and tendons).

Because of the liver's role in generating movement, excessive liver function can result in excessive spontaneous movement. For example, Tourette's syndrome is a neurological disorder that causes spontaneous movement. In TCM, such a clinical presentation would be seen as excessive liver function. Similarly, Qigong practitioners experience spontaneous movement during practice, which could be a result of the liver draining off excess qi. Another example is when you get very angry—what do you do? You start to shake. (I have never seen anyone get so angry that they start to laugh.) This is because the liver is also the seat of the emotion of anger. When you get angry, the liver overactivates and expresses itself through movement.

When the binding and movement structures of the body become weak, this indicates an underfunctioning liver. For example, why is it that a twisted ankle often takes a long time to heal? One reason may be a lack of circulation to the damaged structures. Since the liver adjusts the flow of blood, it is often necessary to strengthen its activity, enabling more blood to flow through the injured area. As noted earlier, practicing the xu sound with an emphasis on the vowel component has a strengthening effect on the liver, so if you sustain an injury to your fascia, ligaments, tendons, or muscles, try practicing the liver Healing Sound in this manner in order to enhance its capacity to facilitate the healing of those structures.

The third function of the liver concerns its relationship to the heart. In TCM theory, a person is seen primarily in terms of the relationships among the different organs. Because of the pattern of the five elements, some organs are directly related to each other. The liver has a very intimate relationship with the heart, because wood directly nurtures fire (and the heart is fire). Therefore, in the alchemical ritual you see that the wood bowl is adjacent to the heart vessel with the flame burning beneath it. When we pour the water into the heart vessel, it symbolizes the liver pouring cooling water into the heart, both soothing the heart and allowing it to heat up the water and turn it into the fluid that, according to TCM, we use for digestion. So, the liver actually initiates all organic processes, and in this very first step, we see the function of the liver as it relates to the heart.

If there is not enough blood for the liver to give to the heart, an excess of heat builds up in the system. This heat manifests as anxiety. In China, when someone goes to a traditional Chinese doctor because of anxiety, the problem is often seen in TCM as blood deficiency, and the doctor prescribes herbs to soothe and enrich the blood in the liver, as was the case with many of the patients I saw while working at a TCM hospital in China. The herbalist would prescribe blood-enriching herbs, and the patient's anxiety would gradually go away.

So, when the heart is overheated, one has anxiety and is "ill at ease." Again, when people are anxious, what do they do? They move around. They have insomnia, and they toss and turn in bed. The liver's function is to cool and soothe the heart, and since the heart is the seat of emotion, consciousness, and awareness, this relieves anxiety. (In TCM, we feel and think with our heart, so in ancient times they used to say, "you have a stupid heart, let's give you a better heart, it improves your intelligence.") Therefore, if one gets anxious, one can practice the consonant part of the xu Healing Sound, and this should help to alleviate some of the anxiety.

The Healing Sounds have existed in the Taoist traditional practice for three thousand years. They are primordial sounds, which the ancient Taoist masters divined from their deep internal experience of nature. Because the sounds are archetypal, they are necessarily trans-cultural and transethnic. For example, I have never seen a mother in any culture try to quiet an overactive, anxious child by yelling, "Hey, hey, hey, hey, hey, quiet down!" Instead, she'll say, "hush" or make the sound "shhh," which are sounds very similar to the liver Healing Sound xu. These sounds serve to calm the anxious child—and remember that the xu sound has a cooling effect. It is the sound of leaves rustling in the springtime wind. When I was in college, one of my poetry teachers came from Iowa, where they grow millions of acres of corn, and he said that if you put your ear to the ground on a very quiet night, you could hear the corn growing. I imagine that this must be much the same sound as xu, the sound of spring.

Truly then, the Healing Sound of xu allows one entry into the profound alchemical practice of Taoism, which is transforming sickness into health, transforming lead into gold. It all begins with a single simple breath. How tragic that we do not see how healing and health rely on the freeing of the breath and the spirit. This idea is reflected in our word *inspiration*.

General Healing Sounds Meditation

Practice the general Healing Sounds meditation as described on pages 48–49. In preparing for the liver meditation, you will want to pay special attention to the following:

- Since liver is associated with the wood element, which tends to generate heat, during the liver meditation you can release excessive heat by gently pressing your thumb to the base of the ring finger.

- In TCM, the liver is also the organ that generates anger and rest-lessness. Since the liver qi/energy extends to the hair, comb your hair with your fingers before and after the liver meditation. This will soothe any feelings of unease that may arise from the liver meditation.

Liver Meditation: Dance of the Bean Sprouts

Is Jack a fool who sold his mother's cow for a handful of beans?
Or does he intuit that beans and plants are the essence of life?

This meditation is based on the liver meridian, which is the path-way for the flow of liver qi through the body. To begin the medita-tion, imagine a small bean beginning to sprout from a crack in the space between the first and second toes of each foot. As the sprouts grow, they slowly creep up your feet and turn inward as if growing up the inside of your calves. As they continue their upward journey along the inside of your knees and thighs, allow a soothing sensation of warmth to spread upward through your thighs to your groin.

Observe the sprouts continuing to grow upward through your torso, branching outward at your waist. Finally, allow the beanstalks to curve back slightly toward your center, ending at the base of your ribs, a few inches below your nipples. The vines have now reached their home, the liver. Imagine the cooling sensation of a light spring breeze gently blowing the plants, and allow this soothing energy to permeate your whole liver.

Let this comforting feeling spread to the rest of your body. If you notice a sudden flash of heat, breathe in and exhale, letting go. Let the heat release from the pores of your skin.

Now imagine the whole bean plant, from the crack between your first and second toes, up through the inside of your legs, con-tinuing through the knees, the thighs, spreading out to the groin, to the sides of the torso, and curving back to the area just below your nipples.

If you notice any spontaneous movement, allow it to happen. If you experience any emotion or physical sensation, allow it to happen.

Breathe in and out deeply three times, using the Himalayan AH sound with each exhalation.

Slowly open your eyes. Inhale. Extend your arms out to the side and push your palms out, exhaling. Breathe in again, and then exhale, pushing your palms up toward the heavens. Finally, inhale and bring your palms to your knees. Exhale and gently press down on your knees. At the same time, very gently shake your spine or any part of your body that you need to shake.

Liver Healing Sound Instruction: XU

Imagine that the couple seated behind you at the movies is providing a running commentary on every scene. Finally, with slight annoyance, you turn around with a finger to your lips and hiss, "Shhhhh." That is the quintessential liver Healing Sound.

Sound Component	Description
Consonant: *Sh*	*Shhhhh* as in hushing a baby.
Vowel: *U*	*U* as in *shoe*, with the oe extended and the rounded mouth of the above hushing sound.
Subvocal wind sound: *Hr*	*Hr* with a breathy nonvocal sound. As if you are blowing a feather off a baby's face, there is only the gentle wind current of your breath without making any noise, or almost like the soft purring of a cat.

Breath Integrals	*Specifics*
Tongue	The sides of the tongue touch the teeth.
Lips	Round them as if to whistle.

Liver Healing Sound Vocal Instruction

The liver Healing Sound xu has three components:

- The consonant *sh* releases the excessive build-up of heat exhaust.
- The vowel *u* strengthens the organ.
- The subvocal wind sound *hr* nourishes the organ.

Before doing the xu sound, begin with the Himalayan AH sound. Repeat the AH sound three times to release the breath and warm up your throat. During the practice of the xu sound, keep the eight breath integrals totally relaxed. As you do the sound, make sure you are not squeezing your lower abdomen to get the sound out: keep it soft, like a baby's belly. Also, make sure that the throat is open, and as you say xu, very gently let the side of your tongue touch the inside surface of your teeth, allowing the air to escape through the center of the tongue. Round the lips slightly, as if you are about to hush someone or whistle (see fig. 4.1).

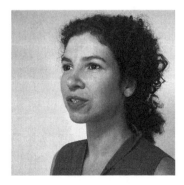

FIGURE 4.1. *XU*

When exhaling with the xu, let out the consonant sound first, and then the vowel, and end with the breathy wind sound of *hr.* This three-part Healing Sound of xu is an important process of letting go of the exhausted air from the lung. Make sure that as you exhale you keep your abdomen soft, without having to push the air out forcefully. Let the air leak out as if from a slowly deflating balloon. Finally, do not forget the wind sound at the end.

Repeat the sound three times. Between each repetition, relax for a moment, breathing naturally for a few cycles.

Liver Healing Sound Movement Instruction

Imagine that you have become the Tree of Life. Suddenly you find that time has slowed down. You are rooted in the soil. Your arms become tree limbs as they slowly stretch up to feed on the honey liquid light of the sun. Spreading your fingers like leaves, you feel the life-giving luminosity stream down to your feet.

The following instruction is given according to a system I have developed in which I label each movement phase with a unique command. This serves as a mnemonic device to help students remember the movements.

- *Gather.* Place one hand on top of the other with the palms on your *dantien,* the Elixir Field, located three finger-widths below the navel, like a sapling with its limbs enfolded, embracing itself (see fig. 4.2).
- *Open.* As you inhale, unfurl and open the palms so that the backs of the hands are touching each other with the fingers pointed down (see fig. 4.3).
- *Arise.* Continuing to inhale, slowly raise the palms to the level of the solar plexus (see fig. 4.4).
- *Extend.* Exhale with the xu sound, as your arms extend out to the sides starting from the shoulder, then the elbow, the wrist, and finally the hands. Make sure the xu sound is synchronized

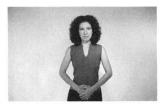

FIGURE 4.2. *Gather*

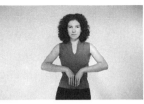

FIGURE 4.3. *Open*

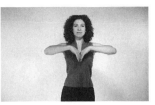

FIGURE 4.4. *Arise*

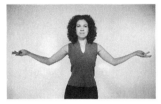

FIGURE 4.5. *Extend*

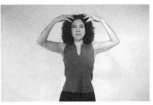

FIGURE 4.6. *Embrace*

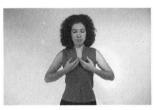

FIGURE 4.7. *Descend*

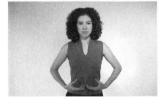

FIGURE 4.8

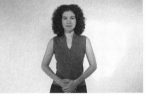

FIGURE 4.9. *Gather*

with the extension of the arms. Continue maintaining this posture as long as you are exhaling the xu sound (see fig. 4.5). This motion is like a young tree growing, its branches reaching out to the sides; your palms are like leaves opening to the heavens, with the thumbs of each hand touching the base of your third finger. Reminder: In the Extend posture, let the xu sound reverberate throughout the entire body, from your fingertips to the roots of your hair. Sing the xu softly, like young leaves unfurling from trees, and never squeeze out the last breath.

- *Embrace.* After finishing the xu sound, inhale, and let your hands gather toward your forehead, with the palms facing you (see fig. 4.6). Imagine you have just released all the exhaustion from the body, and in the embrace, you're gathering in freshness, hope, and vitality. Now allow a full inhalation.

- *Descend.* Exhale and slowly let the palms descend the central line of the body, past the tip of the nose, the heart, and back to the abdomen (see figs. 4.7 and 4.8). As you let your palms softly descend the front of your body, exhale effortlessly, avoiding any unnecessary squeezing of your stomach or neck muscles. Let the energy cascade down the midline of the body; let it pass through the heart and the liver, as if you were a tree gathering its sweet sap from the branches through the trunk back to the roots. Let the sweet sap of your *jing*, your life essence, descend to the abdomen.

- *Gather.* Inhale and embrace the abdomen, with the palms overlapping like two intertwined leaves at the Elixir Field (see fig. 4.9). Pause for a moment and imagine sending soothing light to your liver.

Repeat the sequence three to six times. When you have finished, relax for a moment. Then slowly open your eyes, relax, and stretch out, shaking out your hands. With your fingertips, tap your chest to release any remaining tension.

Refining the Liver Healing Sound Qigong

Make sure the movement and the sound are synchronized. The basic principle of Qigong breathing is that when you extend your arms outward, exhale; when you gather your arms inward toward your body, inhale.

At the Gather phase, close your eyes momentarily to scan the flow of energy within your body. Initially, you might not notice the internal flow of qi. It is a subtle tingling sensation that is sensed internally. Developing this inner sensing cultivates your awareness, and with dedicated practice, you will start to notice subtle changes in your inner landscape. Placing the palms at the dantien—the

Elixir Field, which is an energy nexus for the storage of qi—gathers in the qi from the universe. Energetically, the Elixir Field is shaped like an hourglass lying on its side, bridging the lower back and the front of the abdomen, three finger-widths beneath the navel. Possibly, the early Taoists correlated the Elixir Field with the womb, which has life-generating power. For women in general, it is good to let the qi/energy circulate from the Elixir Field to the rest of the body. Otherwise, a concentration of energy in this region will create too much heat for the female reproductive organs. Since the male sex organs are outside the body, this is not a concern for men.

In overlapping the palms, for women, the right palm should be closest to the body, and for men, the left palm should be closest to the body. This applies to the Gather phase for the rest of the Six Healing Sounds.

During the Descend phase, don't rush and speed up the movement. If you run out of breath, by all means cheat a little with a tiny inhalation in between the long exhalations. Cheating in Qigong is allowed—and recommended! After all, the practice of Qigong is about really getting to get to know your own bodily needs and functions. Don't force your breathing and movements into a rigid pattern.

Healing Sound Story: Don't Cry, Little Fishy

"Don't cry, little fishy, don't cry, don't cry, little fishy, fishh . . . fishhhu," my wife, Janet, sang to our firstborn daughter when she was just two days old.

Janet has a graduate degree in human development. When we were first dating, Janet and I cotaught in a summer arts preschool program. To see her holding our newborn baby and singing this lullaby was a sharp contrast to our academic training. But sometimes one just has to let instinct take over and flow with it. I realized Janet had spontaneously made up a song to lull our baby to sleep. The symbol of a little fishy was very poignant from our experience the previous night.

As new parents, we were astonished at how instinctually our daughter reacted to sounds and smells. The first morning at home, as Janet lay asleep, the baby squirmed about a foot across the bed toward her mother's breast. In our child development studies, we were taught that a newborn does not have any means of locomotion. But apparently the ancient swimming instinct exists in newborns. They also assist in their birth process by literally swimming down the birth canal headfirst in a dolphinlike motion. In Russia, where they experiment with birth in a pool, the newborns emerge from their mothers and start to swim like dolphins.

As our baby slowly drifted off to sleep, Janet's voice lowered to a whisper and stretched the last syllable of the word *fishhhu* into a kind of soothing, wavelike hush.

Suddenly, it dawned on me that the shhhu sound closely resembled the Taoist Healing Sound of xu, a gentle sound to soothe the liver. Perhaps that was how the primal Healing Sounds originated. As our ancestral mothers rocked their babies, they instinctually emitted the xu sound to lull them to sleep. At that instant, Janet's singing connected her to the long line of mothers from the beginning of time.

Healing Sound Story: Luminous Light

Pamela came to me via an urgent call from one of my students, who happened to be her neighbor. Pam lived with her husband in a suburb of New York. She was afraid of traveling and stayed in her local area. Her husband was frantic because Pam began to have seizures and fainting spells after following the instructions in a New Age how-to book on meditation.

When Pam walked into my office, I noticed that her face was bright red and she was slightly overweight. Her breath was short. Her husband was waiting for her outside in the car.

"I was reading daily from this pack of New Age wholistic cards," she said. "One day I picked a card. On it was the instruction, 'Take a moment in your life, sit quietly for ten minutes and concentrate on your breath.' I sat down and started to focus on my breathing, and all of a sudden, I felt this overwhelming heat rush up to my head. My whole body started to shake and I fell backward." Her voice was quivering slightly as she recalled the incident.

"Have you had any prior meditation instruction?" I asked.

"No. I read many books on spiritual subjects," she replied shyly.

"In your case, you have a very unique energy pattern, and that simple breath awareness meditation was counterproductive for you. Your basic energy pattern is one of excessive heat. When you started to focus your attention on your breath, it was as if you had fanned a roaring fire and the flame leaped up. The heat you felt was a direct result of that breath meditation." I spoke gently because I noticed that she was on the verge of tears, as if she had been caught doing something wrong.

"In Taoist practice," I told her, "there are approximately three hundred major meditations. It is crucial that a novice be assigned a meditative process that fits his or her energy and physical pattern. For you, the Luminous Light meditation will help to cool you down and reduce the excessive heat. Furthermore, I will teach you the xu Healing Sound to release excessive fire from your liver."

I asked her to sit in a chair as I placed my palms around her energy field and released the buildup of excessive fire. After ten minutes, her face became less red and soon returned to a normal color. She gave a sigh of relaxation.

"How do you feel?" I asked her.

"Oh, I feel much cooler, and the pressure in my head seems to be less." She sighed again.

"Did you notice the sound you just made?" I gently questioned her.

"Yes, it is like the sound of a teakettle releasing its steam," she replied.

"Yes, you just spontaneously released your steam with the liver xu wind breath. When you go home, do the xu in that breathy, steam-releasing way of sighing, every time you feel the heat start to rise up to your head." I demonstrated the movement of the arms opening to the sides.

Pamela came back in a month and reported with a smile that all the symptoms had gone away.

"One day I was meditating, looking at the light in front of me. Slowly, the light started to get more intense and started to fill the whole room. Then the light expanded toward me, and I felt my body dissolve into the white light. I felt total relaxation and felt that all the excessive heat from my body was released into the light. My body disappeared, but I wasn't scared. Is this normal?" she asked.

"Your experience is a very good indication that you entered into the meditative state. The dissolving into the light is a sign of your mind being in a very rested state. Continue your meditation and Healing Sound, but do not cling to any phenomena. Let any sensations or images come and go without clinging to them," I said, and smiled. I was surprised at her rapid development in the Luminous Meditation.

After a year, Pamela was able to take the train by herself to the city to see me.

"Sometimes, when I am doing the Healing Sound Qigong, I notice that the energy runs up and down along some invisible tubes in my body," she told me after the second year of her study.

"Hmm. Have you ever studied any acupuncture or Chinese medicine?" I asked.

"No, I've never studied anything like that."

"Can you describe the tubes?" I asked.

Pamela indicated the path of the tubes. To my surprise, they exactly matched the Chinese acupuncture liver meridians.

She had discovered this all by herself, intuitively, without any prior study.

Working with Pamela has taught me the lesson of simplicity and spontaneous energy discovery. It has also served as an example of the danger that exists when one tries to learn by oneself, without adequate supervision from a trained teacher. I feel that she is especially gifted and endowed with great inner energy. When she was given the proper instruction, she blossomed.

At the time of this writing, Pamela is in her fifth year of study with me, and now she is tackling her relationship with her father. From my perspective, when one's liver becomes healthy and strong, one can then have enough courage to deal with overbearing forces in one's life.

Perhaps the practice of Qigong and the xu Healing Sound for the liver served as a key to unlock emotional blockage for Pamela. On the other hand, she deserves credit for using these techniques as a key to open her blockage. I have always believed that any technique is a dead thing: only the person has the power to bring it to life.

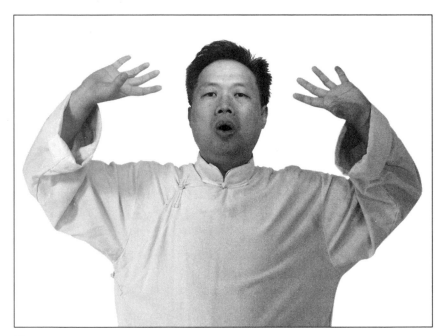

Heart

5

HEART: THE RIVER OF LIFE

Heart shines out like
Solitary moon,
Reflects on a thousand ponds.

WHAT IS the function of the heart? The most obvious function is related to the action of the heart's element, fire. The fire of the heart warms the blood and generates the force behind its distribution throughout the body. In TCM, the heart has the dual functions of warming and pumping the blood. What else does fire do? It illuminates and sheds light on things, so that one can have clear sight and understanding. Therefore, in Chinese medicine, the heart is also the seat of consciousness and is responsible for overseeing cognition and the central nervous system in general. But here is the rub: because it has both a physical and a mental function, this creates tremendous stress for the heart. It is like a single mother who has to work all day and then go home and care for her children. With so much to do, the mother can very easily get overheated, just like the heart.

Thus, the heart is prone to overheating, and when the heart gets overheated, the blood becomes much thicker. When the blood becomes sticky, the circulation gets sluggish, and this may cause blockages throughout the whole cardiovascular system. Sticky blood will cause pathogens and toxins to be stuck inside the various organs such as the liver, the uterus, and the prostate. Moreover, sluggish circulation means that one is not getting nutrients fast enough. It is ironic that while one's blood is so rich one's body can be starving. This overheating of the heart causes a chain reaction that in TCM is believed to be responsible for many sicknesses, such as heart attack, stroke, psychosis, and cancer-related illnesses. From a TCM perspective, high-impact aerobic exercise has a detrimental effect on people who are already stressed out, because their hearts are already overheated. Some people, after a hard day of work, go to the gym and do a high-stress, high-impact aerobic workout to get out their frustrations. From a TCM vantage point, though, this is detrimental. Why? Because the heart will overheat, and if it does, one is in trouble.

Therefore, it is quite obvious from the standpoint of TCM that any mood-altering drugs will harm the heart by causing it to overheat. A drug like cocaine is especially harmful, for it overstimulates the heart, producing a mental state of excess joy and euphoria. Marijuana also affects the heart and circulatory system.

In contrast, the slow, soothing movements and deep breathing of Taiji Quan and Qigong actually help to cool the heart and restore its normal function. In the Six Healing Sounds Qigong, the HO sound has a cooling effect on the heart. So, the next time you run to catch a train and squeeze through the door just before it shuts, with your heart pounding, just take a moment to say HO and see what happens. Just don't do it during Christmas season unless you want to be mistaken for a Santa Claus in training.

The HO sound is also the sound of laughter. Laughter and joy are the universal medicine for sickness. We know that there is strong scientific evidence that laughter and joy improve our immune system's defense against disease. I have always wondered if the Taoist Healing Sound HO is ancient, formalized "laughing therapy." Of course, 2,500 years ago, we did not have the films of the Marx Brothers to help us laugh. However, in the Chinese tradition, there is the Laughing Buddha, who points out to us that the best way of life is that of laughter and humor. In Chinese New Year celebrations, there is a traditional lion dance, in which one sees the lion moving around angry and hungry, because at the end of the year there is not much food. The Laughing Buddha distracts and leads the lion, teasing it out of its anger with his continuous laughter. This dance formalizes the notion that anger can be transformed through the power of laughter. So the next time you have a terrible fight with your partner or a loved one, rather than yelling at each other, try laughing at each other, and I assure you the anger won't last too long. Thus, the Healing Sound of HO, of laughter, gives us a way to transform anger into joy, sickness into health. Our own spontaneous healing starts with the simple sound of laughter.

General Healing Sounds Meditation

Practice the general Healing Sounds meditation as described on pages 48–49. In preparing for the heart Meditation, you will want to pay special attention to the following:

- The heart meridian/energy channel starts at the armpit and ends at the top of the pinkie. Wiggling your pinkies a few times—as if you are plucking an invisible string—will stimulate the heart's qi/energy flow freely along its meridian.

Heart Meditation: Flossing the Cardiovascular System

Thread a tiny light through the heart chambers and its rivulets.
Cleanse them of all debris.
Let the river of life rejuvenate its free flow.

Sit at ease. If you are sitting on a chair, sit at the edge, with your feet flat on the floor. Place your palms on your knees. Let your eyes gently close. Allow the tip of your tongue to roll down and touch your lower palate.

Visualize your heart in the center of your chest. The heart is divided into two chambers, the right and the left. Inhale and imagine a tiny thread of light starting from the right heart chamber, flowing with the blood out to the lungs. Exhale. Feel warmth spreading through the lungs as the light reaches out to their surface. Inhale deeply and let the oxygen from the lungs diffuse into the blood.

Continue the journey, and let the light return from the lungs back to your left heart chamber. When the light returns to your heart, feel a burst of joy, with a slight contraction in your heart.

Exhale. Now imagine that the light from the left chamber of your heart overflows into the central artery. As the light moves down the artery and into your abdominal region, let it clean out any debris that it encounters along the way.

Inhale and allow the light to travel down to both kidneys. Breathe naturally for a few breaths. With each inhalation, fill the kidneys with light and soothing warmth. Let the kidneys relax and then contract slightly in a rhythmic pumping motion. Continue breathing naturally. Imagine the light descending from the kidneys through the urinary tract and into the bladder. Allow the light to cleanse any debris in the urinary tract and the bladder. From there, feel the warm light moving down the insides of your thighs and legs. Let the light descend all the way down to your toes.

Now imagine the light returning up from the toes, traveling up the backs of your legs as you inhale. Again, imagine that the light is unlocking any blockages along the way. Feel the smoothness of the light within the veins. Exhale and let the light pause momentarily at the lymph nodes in the groin area. As you continue breathing softly, you may feel a soft warmth or even a slight ticklish feeling in the area.

Inhale deeply. Pull up the perineum, and gently let the light surge up through the tailbone and up the lower back. Exhale. Inhale again and let the light go up the middle back, the upper back, through the neck and into your brain. Breathe naturally for a few seconds, and then let the light circulate up to the crown of your head, down behind your eyes, behind your nose, and finally descend into your heart. Take in a deep breath. From the heart, let the light radiate out to the universe in a thousand rays. As you silently exhale, a profound, joyous sound of HO, like laughter, emanates outward, rippling infinitely into the universe, sharing your joy and light with all sentient beings. Breathe naturally, continuing to allow the light to radiate out.

After a while, slowly come back, gradually allow your eyes to open, inhale, and gently raise your hands as if you were yawning. Exhale with the sound HO. Inhale, stretch your arms out to the side, and exhale. Inhale again, let the arms drop down and press your palms on your knees, straighten your spine, and exhale.

Heart Healing Sound Instruction: HO

Sound Component	Description
Consonant: *H*	*H* has no sound; it functions to release heat.
Vowel: *O*	*O* is like the foghorn of an old steamship.
Subvocal wind sound: *Hhho*	*Hhho* is a breathy nonvocal sound, as if you are warming up your hands on a cold winter morning.

Breath Integral for the Heart

Breath Integrals	Specifics
Tongue	The tip of the tongue touches the bottom of the palate.
Lips	Make your lips full and round as if you are blowing a smoke ring.

Heart Healing Sound Vocal Instruction

Before performing the heart sound itself, it is good to warm up with the Himalayan AH sound. Imagine that after ten long, grueling years working as a dishwasher in a restaurant, you finally get enough money to fulfill your one dream, which is to lug a hundred-pound oxygen tank over thousands of miles to see the Himalayan Mountains. When you finally arrive in the Himalayas, you see the mountains and you say AH. Was it worth it? You say AH. You start to feel good. And you inhale again and say AH.

The Himalayan sound allows us to warm up our eight breath integrals (diaphragm, ribs, lungs, bronchi, throat and larynx, soft palate, tongue, and jaw and lips). So when you exhale, let the diaphragm come up, pushing up the heart and helping it to pump out the blood. Drop your jaw and soften the back of your throat and say AH. Repeat at least three times.

The Healing Sound for the heart, HO, has three components: a consonant sound, a vowel sound, and a wind sound. The consonant sound is an *h,* but actually it has no sound. The role of the consonant is that it helps to release excessive build up of heat in the heart.

The vowel sound is an *o.* To make this, round the lips and touch the tip of the tongue to the bottom of the mouth. Try to open the mouth as wide as possible without tension (see fig. 5.1). The HO

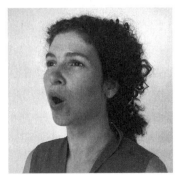

FIGURE 5.1. *HO*

sounds like an old steamship's whistle blowing for departure. The vowel sound serves to strengthen the organ.

The third component, the wind sound, is a subvocal sounding of the HO. It is like blowing onto your hands to warm them up when it is freezing outside. This has a function of nourishing the organ. When exhaling with the HO sound, let the consonant *h* sound out first, then the vowel *o,* and end with the breathy wind sound of *hhho.*

All three parts of the Healing Sound HO are important in the process of letting out exhausted air from the lungs. Make sure that as you exhale, you keep your abdomen soft, without contracting it to push the breath out. Lay your palms on your abdomen, and as you say HO, jiggle it like a bowl of jelly. Let the air leak out, as if from a slowly deflating balloon. While you are chanting the HO sound, allow the back of your throat and the back of your head to vibrate. This will help to release any blockages in the sinuses and inner ear. You can place your hands on the back of your head as you say the HO sound.

Simply doing the HO sound without any accompanying movements can still have healing benefits for the heart. With daily practice, you will start to develop your own sense of how to do the Healing Sound. Listen to the sound and sense your breath, making sure that you are doing it without any tension. The foundation of the Healing Sounds lies in freeing the breath, and the sound therefore gives you feedback as to whether you are tight, tense, or out of breath. If you can say the sound HO for only a short duration, you are out of breath. In time, with practice, the breath will lengthen.

Heart Healing Sound Movement Instruction

- *Gather.* Begin with your hands folded one over the other at the Elixir Field, located three finger-widths below the navel. This entices the fire qi of the heart to gather in the belly. In alchemical terms, this is called lowering heart fire to heat up kidney water. Thus, this process generates warmth and internal steam to empower the internal circulation of the endocrine fluids, the kidney water (see fig. 5.2).
- *Open.* Inhale and separate your hands to one fist space apart and unfurl the palms, turning them to face upward. Imagine that

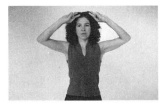

FIGURE 5.2. *Gather*

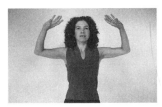

FIGURE 5.3. *Open*

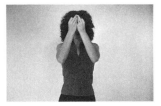

FIGURE 5.4

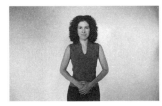

FIGURE 5.5

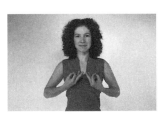

FIGURE 5.6. *Arise*

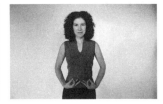

FIGURE 5.7. *Emerge*

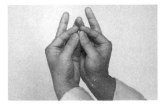

FIGURE 5.8. *Bloom*

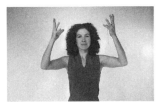

FIGURE 5.9

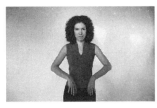

FIGURE 5.10. *Embrace*

your hands become a young lotus flower bud: touching the tips of your thumb, pinkie, and index finger together shapes the hands into the lotus mudra, which has a calming effect on the central nervous system (see figs. 5.3, 5.4, and 5.5).

- *Arise.* Continuing to inhale, imagine that the hands are like a lotus blossom surfacing and emerging from the bottom of a pond, and let them gently rise up from the abdomen to the heart (see fig. 5.6).

- *Emerge.* Continuing to inhale, imagine your hands in the lotus mudra like a blossom breaking through from the water to the air. With your hands still in mudra, bring your hands up in front of your throat, then nose, and finally to your forehead. At the forehead, feel the warmth of your fingertips as they lightly touch your head (see fig. 5.7).

- *Bloom.* Let your fingers open out like petals. Unfurl your palms like sunflowers, and stretch your arms out to the side, with your palms facing the heavens. Simultaneously, exhale with the sound HO (see figs. 5.8 and 5.9). At this point, envision that you are gently holding a soft pillow above your head. In certain esoteric

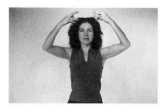

FIGURE 5.11

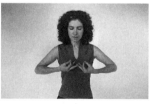

FIGURE 5.12. *Full Moon*

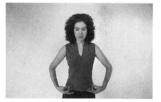

FIGURE 5.13. *Descend*

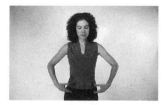

FIGURE 5.14. *Gather*

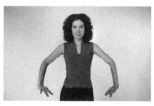

FIGURE 5.15

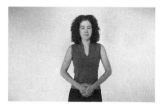

FIGURE 5.16

Buddhist practices, one visualizes holding the feet of the Buddha. Allow the sound of HO to resonate throughout your whole body from head to toe. (Note: If you feel any discomfort or have any shoulder problems, do not raise the palms higher than the level of your shoulders.) Reminder: You can stay in the Bloom posture for the full duration of the HO sound. The Bloom posture has a special curative effect in opening the heart. This effect is due to the stretching of the heart meridians along the underside of the arms in this position.

- *Embrace.* After finishing exhalation with the HO sound, inhale and gather your fingertips together at the forehead into lotus mudra, just like a lotus blossom closing in the evening (see figs. 5.10 and 5.11).
- *Full Moon.* Continue to inhale and let your hands slowly descend from the forehead down to your heart. At this point, imagine that your palms are like flower petals closing up for the night (see fig. 5.12). Pause for a moment to sense your heart. Try to soften the heart with the imagery of a full moon shining within it. The moonlight illuminates the heart with its soft translucent beams. (Note: you may suddenly hear the throbbing of the heart. It is quite normal and will soon pass as the heart readjusts itself.)
- *Descend.* Exhale, letting the palms descend to the level of your navel, like a lotus seed sinking to the bottom of a pond (see fig. 5.13).
- *Gather.* Let the hands make a circular path, as if you are playing with the water by making a small ripple. Fold them one over the other at the Elixir Field (see fig. 5.14, 5.15, and 5.16). Take a moment to let your breath return to its normal pace. If you find at any point in the exercise that your breath is tight or tense, or if continuously inhaling or exhaling is too difficult, break up the breaths and take shorter ones in between. Always make sure that your breathing is natural and easy. This is also a good time to sense your body to verify the effect of the Healing Sounds. Notice whether there is any incremental shift or

change in your posture, breath, balance, or emotions. Notice whether you feel a sense of joyous tranquillity. There is no right way to feel. Just spread out your senses like tentacles to every part of your body, mind, and spirit. Eventually, you may begin to feel the more subtle flow of energy, qi, moving in your energy meridians. At the moment after finishing a single Healing Sounds cycle, it is very beneficial to let the healing effect occur without rushing into the next cycle. This moment is like the silence at the end of Beethoven's Ninth Symphony. Too often, the audience will rush to applaud without savoring this eternal moment of silence.

Repeat the process three to six times. After even a single repetition, you will find that the movement will get smoother and the breath more at ease because your body, joints, and energy pathways will have been opened. With each repetition, see if you can expand your awareness and sense more details in your movements.

Refining the Heart Healing Sound Qigong

In the Bloom posture, spread your fingers apart to further stretch the heart vessel, which runs from the pinkie to the armpit. In the Full Moon posture, seeing the full moon at the heart is one of the best meditations for healing both insomnia and anxiety. You can stay in the Full Moon posture as long as you wish. Just breathe normally. The heart Healing Sound is a powerful sound that can open the door to our inner landscape and its internal energy flow.

Healing Sound Story: **Mo Gu Gai Pan**

Whenever my children had any sort of painful accident—bumping their knees, jamming their fingers—they would come to me for comfort.

"*Mo Gu Gai Pan, Mo Gu Gai Pan . . .*" I held on to their hurt and pain while chanting these words. At the same time, I would stroke the area as if physically pulling out the pain and then pretend to throw it out the window. Usually, they would feel much better after such "magic."

"What is that chant, Daddy?" they would ask me.

"Oh, it is a sacred chant that I learned as a young man from a Taoist magician," I would say.

One summer, my daughter Lingji was invited to dance her own choreography at Jacob's Pillow Dance Festival. It was a duet entitled *Lineage,* and I was her dance partner. Just a few days before the concert, I had bitten my tongue badly while eating a rock-hard bagel. For the entire concert, I could hardly speak because my tongue was extremely swollen. Every day I would practice Qigong and the heart Healing Sound of HO to reduce the pain and hasten the healing process. According to TCM principles, the tongue is the bud of the heart. After a few days, the swelling had gone down and I could eat without too much difficulty.

On the last night after the final performance, our whole family decided to celebrate and went to a Chinese restaurant for dinner.

As they started to read the Chinese menu, my daughters made the shocking discovery that *Mo Gu Gai Pan* is actually a dish of chicken with mushrooms!

"Oh, Daddy, they have *Mo Gu Gai Pan* here! All these years, we have been chanting a Chinese dish!" they said incredulously.

"Oh, that must be the chant I learned as a young man while serving food in a Chinese restaurant," I laughed. It was wonderful, after so many years, to have them finally discover my little secret.

"Then I should order the *Mo Gu Gai Pan* to heal my tongue," I continued.

As I ate the *Mo Gu Gai Pan,* my tongue felt much better, and by the next day the swelling had gone down completely. Part of me knew it was due to the saltiness of the dish, but another part of me was amazed that the chant did have healing power.

"From now on, if you ever feel sad or hurt, you can always order *Mo Gu Gai Pan* and it will make you feel better," I told my children afterward.

I hope that wherever they go, may their hurts and pains be easily relieved by the simple chant, *Mo Gu Gai Pan*.

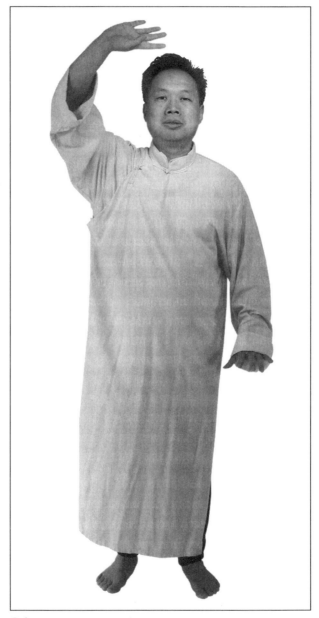

Spleen

6

SPLEEN:
THE MOTHER EARTH

Earth absorbs all lives
And returns them as flowers, fruits, and blessings.
My bare foot kisses the moist earth with each step.
How wonderful to feel the earth lifting me up,
As I stretch out my arms toward the stars.

IN TCM, the spleen and pancreas are considered as a single organ, so when a Chinese doctor refers to the spleen, he or she is also referring to the pancreas. What are the function and qualities of the spleen? The spleen is represented by the element earth. The three most important aspects of the spleen's function are transforming food into nourishment, moisturizing the body, and helping the body regenerate after sickness or trauma.

The spleen's major qualities are sweetness, earthiness, and absorption. In the alchemical ritual of cocoa, the yellow bowl containing cocoa powder represents the spleen, so if you want to remember the qualities of the spleen, just remember the characteristics of cocoa powder.

Spleen qi is pervasive. The spleen is like the vastness of earth. It is like the center of a spider's web. Its influence extends outward to every aspect of your organs' functioning. From the moment you are born, the spleen directly influences every activity in your body.

The primary function of the spleen is to transform food into nourishment. In other words, the spleen is in charge of changing what we eat into sustenance that the body can absorb. Additionally, the spleen governs and directs the distribution of the nutrients throughout the body. Think of it as the farmer's wife, who must prepare meals for her family and also for all the farmhands. This is the spleen: the hearth, the mother, and the cook.

Another function of the spleen is to moisturize the burning heart. Without the moisture of the spleen, the heart's fire can easily overheat. This can induce symptoms such as hypertension (high blood pressure), insomnia, and in some extreme cases, withering of the heart muscles.

Finally, the spleen, just like the earth, has the miraculous power of regeneration. In order for us to recuperate from serious sickness, the spleen has to function properly. It is similar to the aftermath of a volcanic eruption, where, despite the trauma of the eruption, the earth can regenerate and transform barren soil so that it is soon teeming with life again. Similarly, recuperation from sickness relies on the health and the strength of the spleen.

For example, cancer patients who are undergoing chemotherapy very often lose their appetite. In TCM, loss of appetite is considered a hindrance to the healing process. So in most cases, Chinese doctors would supplement the chemotherapy treatment with herbs to improve the patient's appetite and digestive function. One of the most commonly prescribed herbs is hawthorn berry, and we now know that hawthorn berry not only contains a large amount of vitamin C but also is very rich in digestive enzymes.

During my internship at a hospital in China, one of my TCM professors taught me a very simple rule of thumb for determining which patients in the cancer ward would survive another day. I was expecting him to say that he used something highly esoteric, like pulse diagnosis, urine smelling, or iridology, but he said, "Just look at their food cart after lunch. Is the bowl of rice empty? Did they eat all the food?"

That was it—what indicates whether a patient will survive for another day is whether he or she has an appetite. He told me he had never seen a patient who was about to die eat a good meal. Accordingly, in many cases, as a patient starts to recuperate, the appetite improves. So, when you start to feel sick—let's say that you have a bad case of Hong Kong flu—you will have no appetite. However, as soon as you start to feel better, food suddenly smells good again and you want to eat. That is a sure sign that you are getting better. Taking this into account, most Chinese families will bring delicious delicacies to their loved ones in the hospital. With a bit of guilt, I must admit that I tasted some of the best dishes offered by my patients. What a wonderful way for the patient's family to get involved and also reduce hospital costs.

Now, the above idea applies only to recovering patients. Because of our habit of overeating, and the abundance of cheap food in the developed countries of the Western Hemisphere, many people overstress their digestive system by choking it with excessive food that is not digested and becomes putrid and rotten in the intestines.

This in turn, according to TCM, causes phlegm (cholesterol) in the arteries, leading to heart attack or stroke. This kind of phlegm blockage can also turn into various forms of autoimmune disease, which are internally generated sicknesses, partly due to our own excessive action and self-abusive behavior. (In TCM, a majority of these diseases are attributed to phlegm blockage from habitual overeating.)

Our American culture often encourages overeating—eating for fun. Down the street from where we live in Chelsea's old flower district, we have a wonderful donut shop, and my wife, Janet, goes there from time to time to buy a half-dozen donuts. This donut shop offers a real deal: if you buy a half-dozen donuts, you get another half-dozen for only a dollar. The workers at the shop are always amazed that Janet only wants one half-dozen and not the better deal.

"Why not get another half-dozen for just a dollar?" they ask her.

She simply laughs and pats her stomach. "Oh, but those six 'bonus' donuts would end up costing much more than a dollar," she replies.

In other words, there's no such thing as a free donut. You will have to pay later, maybe when you are stretched on the surgeon's table having a triple coronary artery bypass. So say "pass" to all those 99-cent burger-and-French-fry deals—they might be cheap, but their cost is dear. Cheap junk food will choke the very life out of us.

The ideal of a healthy spleen can be summed up by the Buddha's description of the right effort in meditation: when one plays a stringed instrument, the strings must be neither too tight nor too loose. So, don't become such a glutton that your veins and arteries become blocked, but don't diet to such excess that your body becomes withered and dried up. In women, for instance, excessive weight loss can often result in infertility. Of course, there may be other factors involved in eating disorders, such as genetic and psychological components that can push the body to the extremes of obesity and anorexia. Those cases require specific medical remedies that are beyond the scope of this book.

FU is the healing sound for the spleen. How does FU activate the function of the spleen? One crucial component is our tongue. When you let the tongue float freely in the middle of the mouth while vocalizing the FU sound, the vibration of the tongue stimulates and energizes the activity of the spleen, which starts to secrete its digestive juices, normalizing digestive function. No wonder after a few minutes of doing the FU sound many practitioners experience a feeling of fullness. Therefore, the practice of the FU sound can help us avoid snacking out of habit, thus bringing our eating habits back into a healthy balance.

So, when doing the FU sound, make sure the tongue is not touching any part of your mouth. This is difficult, because we are not used to having our tongue floating freely in the space of the mouth. When you try to do that, what do you discover? Suddenly, you have become very wise, because it is almost impossible to speak when your tongue is in the free-floating position, and you begin to listen a lot more. So when people say, "Hold your tongue," they forget to add "freely in your mouth!" Holding your tongue floating freely in your mouth is the essence of the FU Healing Sound—and perhaps even the road to wisdom.

Another way in which the FU sound assists the spleen is via the buzzing of the lips. This serves to vibrate our entire digestive tract, stimulating its activity. This is because the lips are at one end of the digestive system, which is basically a long tube that includes the lips, mouth, esophagus, stomach, small intestine, large intestine, and rectum. When the lips are loose and you say the FU sound, the vibrations are sent along the whole length of the digestive tract, stimulating the small blood vessels and villae of the intestines, and "shaking out" blockages.[1]

In order to allow this tube to vibrate and buzz, it is very important that you keep the lips very soft and loose. This is the opposite of how most of us usually hold them, which is quite tightly. If you tend to clench your jaw, try practicing keeping your lips loose. This will relax all your facial nerves and muscles and can also have the minor benefit of healing a temporomandibular joint problem.

What are the uses of the FU Healing Sound in terms of its effect on the spleen? As I mentioned earlier, in the TCM model, eating disorders are considered a malfunction of the spleen. Therefore in China, when you overeat, they do not schedule you for liposuction or stomach stapling. Instead they give you herbs or prescribe the spleen Healing Sound in order to help the spleen return to normal, and often you suddenly no longer feel the need to eat compulsively.

Another use of the FU Healing Sound is to dry up overwetness of the spleen, a common pathology of the organ. Just as a flood washes away the earth and can cause a landslide, a common symptom of overflooding of the spleen is local or systemic edema (swelling). The FU Healing Sound enables the evaporation and expulsion of excess fluid, the latter of which is accomplished by stimulating and opening the pores of the skin. Evaporation is enhanced by the free floating of the tongue during the FU sound.

According to TCM, a further situation in which the FU sound may be of benefit is for women who are unable to menstruate because they have depleted their spleen's transformative and nourishing function. The kidneys (the endocrine system) have thus lost their supplier for reproductive hormones. This may occur in female athletes who overwork their bodies or women who diet excessively and become anorexic: they no longer menstruate and therefore cannot reproduce. What's more, it can take those women a long time, even a few years, to recover their normal hormonal cycle (if it is recoverable), because they have damaged the spleen's function of nourishment and transformation of food. There is a practice done by many Buddhist nuns, where they fast until they no longer menstruate. However, their fasting is accomplished by spontaneous cessation of hunger. Many of the nuns report that they are not hungry, so they no longer need to take in food. This is due to a fundamental shift in their mental state and physiology through the practice of meditation and Qigong. For when the mind, heart, and body are in a state of bliss and tranquillity, one no longer requires excessive energy. It is as if one can absorb enough sustenance just by breathing air, drinking water, and soaking up sunlight. So the nuns' fasting is actually a healthy and profound spiritual practice of cutting through the web of desires. Their prolonged fast is a direct result of their lifelong, arduous spiritual cultivation and should not be attempted by anyone else without proper guidance. On the other hand, for a laywoman who is trying to recover from the sort of spleen depletion mentioned above, the Healing Sound of FU will stimulate the spleen's function and assist in restoring the normal cycle of menstruation.

Finally, one can use the FU sound to aid recovery after any sort of illness, especially when one has lost one's appetite. Here, the FU sound helps to strengthen the spleen's recuperative functions by restoring the patient's appetite for food—and for life itself.

General Healing Sounds Meditation

Practice the general Healing Sounds meditation as described on pages 48–49. In preparing for the spleen meditation, you will want to pay special attention to the following:

- Prior to the spleen meditation, gently tap the Leg Three Mile acupressure point (ST-36), located on the outer shin just below the knee. This stimulates the spleen qi/energy to stream down the leg to the toes.

Spleen Meditation

Earth moves in a glacial tempo, dancing in step with sun, moon, and stars. Feel the movement of earth carrying you across the infinite span of galaxies.

Imagine that you are like a sandstone statue, sitting in deep stillness on top of a mountain. As you look out at the far horizon, you see the great expanse of the whole earth beneath you; you see the rich, dark soil of the fertile earth teeming with life. Take a deep breath in, and experience the vastness of the earth as it spreads everywhere. This is the ground of our existence.

For a thousand years, this sandstone statue has stood on top of the mountain, until one day, it cracks—and fissures open along the outer sides of your big toes. Imagine that a warm, golden light fills the space of the fissures. Slowly, the fissures move up along the inside edges of your feet, going along your ankles and up the insides of your knees. Suddenly, you feel a sense of potential movement now that there is space in the statue. As the fissures rise up further along the insides of your thighs, you may feel a ticklish sensation, like a small ant climbing up your leg. Resist the urge to scratch. Continue to let the golden light fill up the space created by the

fissures. Let the fissures continue up the front of your body, cracking further up into your torso, until they are right under your
breasts, at which time they move out to the sides, stopping just
under your armpits.

Enjoy the spaciousness created along the length of both fissures.
Fill them with golden light, and with each breath, let the golden
light become more and more brilliant, as if you were a stone egg
cracking open and the inner essence of your light being were
emerging. Feel sweet nectar drop from the roof of your mouth to
the center of your tongue. Swallow the nectar, letting its moisture
run down from your throat into your spleen, which is located just
beneath your left breast. Very gently, smile to your spleen, and
silently make the sound of FU, to soothe and comfort it. Feel your
spleen, feel your stomach, and feel your whole digestive system unfolding, unfurling, like rich fertile soil covering the entire earth.

Slowly come back, take a deep breath in, and put your palms together in front of your heart. Slowly exhale and stretch your arms
out to the side. Yawn if you need to. Inhale, reach up to the heavens,
and exhale. Finally, inhale, and place your palms on your knees,
stretch your spine upward as you press your palms down, slowly
rolling your shoulders as you do so.

Spleen Healing Sound Instruction: FU

Sound Component	Description
Consonant: *F*	*F* functions to release heat. Its consonant sounds like cooling a spoonful of hot soup.
Vowel: *U*	*U* is like the foghorn on an old steamship.
Subvocal wind sound: *Fff*	*Fff* is a breathy nonvocal sound like the soft sigh of a breeze, a trailing-off of the FU sound as you come to the end of your breath.

Breath Integrals	Specifics
Tongue	It should float freely in the middle of the mouth.
Mouth shape	Lips gently pull back as if you are blowing on hot soup to cool it, keeping the lips loose so that they can vibrate.

Spleen Healing Sound Vocal Instruction

Again, warm up with the Himalayan AH sound. Imagine that it has been wintertime for five months. The earth is bleak and frozen, the subway is not running, and the only thing that is running is take-out service from restaurants. Then, at last, warm weather arrives. You go out into the sunshine and the sky is finally blue. And you take a deep breath and you say AH. If one breath is not enough, inhale another breath deep into your lungs and say AH. After five months you deserve as many AHs as you need.

When practicing the Healing Sounds, be aware that they are nothing more than simple, natural exhalations that are done without any tension. Make certain that you keep the eight breath integrals in a state of relaxation throughout the practice. For the FU sound, keep the diaphragm free from tension. The diaphragm functions very much like a rubber band: during inhalation, it stretches taut, and in exhalation, it retracts without effort. As the diaphragm releases, it floats high up under the ribs and touches the base of the heart. This rising up during exhalation gives the spleen and stomach room to expand after they were compressed during inhalation. One of the crucial aspects of the FU breath is enhancing the diaphragm's motion to massage your spleen and other organs.

Also, in particular for the FU Healing Sound, the tongue should float freely in the middle of the mouth. Finally, keep the lips loose so that they can vibrate, as if you are about to give a very soft, wet kiss to a loved one (see fig. 6.1).

The FU Healing Sound has three components—the consonant,

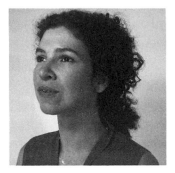

FIGURE 6.1. *FU*

the vowel, and the wind sound. The consonant is the sound *f*, and it allows you to release the excessive buildup of heat exhaust in the spleen. The vowel sound of FU is the sound *u*, and it serves to strengthen the organ. The subvocal wind sound nourishes the organ and is the sound your vibrating lips make when you blow air through them, such as when you are trying to make a baby laugh or imitating the sound of a propeller plane in flight.

When making the FU sound, let the *f* consonant sound come out first, then the *u* vowel sound, and then end with the breathy wind sound. Keep the tongue floating freely in the mouth. Let the lips buzz loosely. You will notice that if your lips are loose and soft, there will be a pocket of air between your lips and your gums. If you do the FU sound correctly, it will sound almost like a foghorn, very soothing.

Back in my college days, my roommate had a girlfriend who grew up near a seaport. As a child she would fall asleep to the low, soulful sound of foghorns. After she moved to New York City, she couldn't get to sleep. Sometimes in the middle of the night, when she stayed over with my roommate, I'd hear the deep rumbling of this soulful sound and think, "What is a foghorn doing here in a basement apartment?" Then I'd dream of being with whales in the deep blue sea. One morning, my roommate sheepishly told me in private that he had to imitate the sound of the foghorn to lull his girlfriend to sleep. Such sweet tenderness.

Spleen Healing Sound Movement Instruction

The image of the spleen Healing Sound movement is of mountains, clouds, and a tumbling stream. The direction of this movement is simultaneously upward and downward. Imagine that your two hands are different elements, one hand moving up toward the heavens like the rising clouds, and the other hand going down toward the earth like a falling stream. Remember to keep your breath soft and your shoulders loose, and do not strain your back.

- *Gather.* To begin, overlap the palms at the Elixir Field, three finger-widths below the navel. Allow warmth from the palm to emanate to the spleen and stomach. Warming the digestive organs enhances their ability to digest food (see fig. 6.2).

- *Arise.* Inhale and slowly raise the palms, folded together like the wings of a swan, from the abdomen, to the heart (see figs. 6.3 and 6.4). This gesture of placing both hands folded at the heart is an expression of sincerity. Sincerity is the characteristic of the spleen.

- *Diverge.* Exhale with the sound of FU. Your two hands separate and move in opposite directions. Raise the right hand up toward the heavens, like a soft cloud, with the palm facing the sky. Simultaneously, the left hand moves downward toward the earth like a falling stream, with the palm facing the ground (see figs. 6.5 and 6.6). If you have any shoulder problems and cannot raise

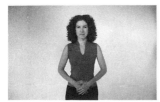 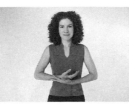 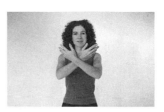

FIGURE 6.2. *Gather*   FIGURE 6.3. *Arise*   FIGURE 6.4

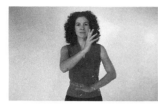

FIGURE 6.5. *Diverge*

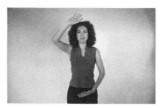

FIGURE 6.6

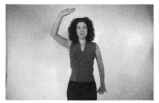

FIGURE 6.7. *Heaven and Earth*

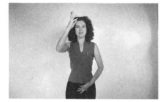

FIGURE 6.8. *Enfold*

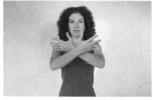

FIGURE 6.9

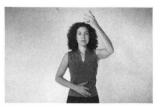

FIGURE 6.10. *Diverge*

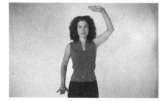

FIGURE 6.11. *Heaven and Earth*

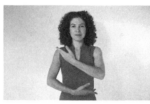

FIGURE 6.12. *Enfold*

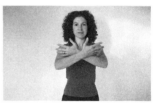

FIGURE 6.13

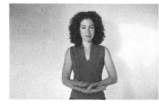

FIGURE 6.14. *Descend*

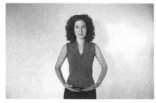

FIGURE 6.15

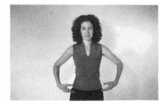

FIGURE 6.16. *Gather*

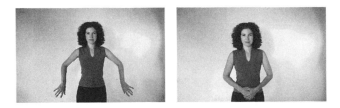

FIGURE 6.17   FIGURE 6.18

your arm above a certain point, just do as much as you can without forcing any movement or causing any discomfort.

- *Heaven and Earth.* Continue exhaling with the FU sound, and stretch the right (cloud) palm directly above your head. At the same time, stretch your left (earth) palm to the level of your thigh (see fig. 6.7). The upward movement of the right palm brings nutrients to the brain and lung from the spleen and stomach organs. The downward movement of the left palm helps to eliminate wastes by transporting them to the large intestine. Maintain this Heaven and Earth posture for the full duration of the FU sound. Feel the sound vibrating in both palms. Make sure the shoulder is not hunched up and the right upper elbow is slightly bent. Feel the opposing stretch between the two palms like bread dough being elongated.

- *Enfold.* Inhale and let the right palm slowly descend to your heart. At the same time, let the left palm slowly rise up and cross the right palm at the heart. Return back to the folded-wings posture of a swan (see figs. 6.8 and 6.9). At this juncture, the right arm overlaps the left arm. The left arm is closest to the body.

- *Diverge.* Exhale with the sound of FU. Your two hands start to diverge and separate in opposite directions. Raise the left hand up toward the heavens like a soft cloud, with the palm facing the sky. Simultaneously, the right hand moves downward toward the earth like a falling stream, with the palm facing the ground (see fig. 6.10).

- *Heaven and Earth.* Continue exhaling with the FU sound, and stretch the left (cloud) palm directly above your head. At the same time, stretch your right (earth) palm to the level of your thigh (see fig. 6.11). This is an exact mirror image of the previous Heaven and Earth posture, with the hands reversing their positions. As you perform this movement with the sound, see if you experience a vibration in the fingertips.

- *Repeat.* Repeat the sequence of Enfold, Diverge, and Heaven and Earth for each palm up to three times.

- *Enfold.* Inhale and let the cloud palm slowly descend to your heart. At the same, let the earth palm at the thigh to slowly rise and cross the other palm at the heart. Return to the folded-wings posture of a swan (see figs. 6.12 and 6.13).

- *Descend.* To finish, exhale and let the hands descend like falling leaves down to the abdomen, three inches below the navel (see figs. 6.14 and 6.15). Take a brief pause and let the qi settle down to the dantien, the Elixir Field.

- *Gather.* Inhale and unfurl the hands outward as if they are making a small rippling motion. Overlap the hands at the Elixir Field (see figs. 6.16, 6.17, and 6.18). Rest in stillness and send internal feelers in the body to assess the effect of the spleen Healing Sound.

Refining the Spleen Healing Sound Qigong

Since the spleen controls the muscular system, the spleen Healing Sound Qigong is one of the most physically demanding of all the Six Healing Sounds. I advise beginning students to approach the spleen practice in baby steps, to move in such a way as to avoid unnecessary shoulder pain. For example, it may be better to raise the arm no higher than the neck level, with the hand in front of the face. Practicing in such a modified way, one can still gain benefits from the Qigong. In time, as the shoulder becomes freer, the arm will naturally lift above the head. I have worked with students who practiced in such modified way and they still gained health benefits. Remember, if the shoe doesn't fit, cut a hole in it. When the Qigong form is too difficult, reduce the range of motion.

With each repetition, always approach the movements with a sense of freshness. Just as the heart beats in a nonrepetitive pattern, nature never repeats itself.

Healing Sound Story: At the Great Shanghai Dumpling House

After our regular morning Qigong class, we would take our teacher out for dumplings, right next to Confucius Plaza in New York's Chinatown. I had figured out that Sifu (the Chinese word for teacher) would sometimes give us some of the most profound teachings during a meal. There is something sacred about sitting around a dining table with a Chinese teacher.

"Ouch!" one of the Western students cried out as he bit into a scalding-hot soup dumpling.

"Ah, you have to blow it gently first to cool it down in your spoon." Sifu started to blow with a soft breathy sound of "Fuuuuuu." I glanced around to see if my classmates had caught the teaching, but they were all too absorbed in eating their dumplings to notice how

Sifu had just revealed the Healing Sound for the spleen. I discreetly jotted it down in my little notebook.

"See, if you blow gently like this, 'Fuuuu,' it will cool the dumpling and make it taste better," he added. I wrote in my notes, "The FU sound will prepare one's digestive system to cool and absorb the food, therefore making the dumpling taste better." In my fifteen years of studying with Sifu, most of his teachings had been off the cuff, just like that day.

Just then, a waiter arrived and served us another steaming pot of dumplings. Sifu looked up and smiled, pointing to the waiter. "You should all get to know Mr. Chang. He is a great Taoist master." We all pushed back our chairs to stand and bow slightly to the middle-aged man with the bright eyes.

"Oh, your teacher is too kind. I am just a simple man. Now, your master is truly a great Taoist with incredible skills," he replied.

"Old Chang, no use to hide now. Why don't you tell my students the story of how you came to America?" Sifu invited him to sit with us.

"Well, if you have a bit of time to waste, I will tell you my own personal experience." He remained standing.

"Yes, please. Will you give us a teaching?" I knew that a student must ask for a teaching formally.

"Being poor, with no money to fly on a plane, I decided the best way to come to America was to work on a tanker. I worked as the cook for the crew. After we had been at sea for a fortnight, a huge typhoon developed during the night. The captain asked everyone, the crew and even the cooking staff, to help to secure the cargo on deck. I wore a life jacket just to be safe. The waves were terrifying. They were like black mountains that loomed up and crashed on the deck. Luckily, the ship was very solidly built." At that moment, the kitchen bell rang. Mr. Chang went to get our other dishes.

After he came back, Mr. Chang continued. "Having been trained in the martial arts, despite the storm I was able to walk without falling down. I noticed one of the crew was having some difficulty in securing the cargo. As I went to help him, all of a sudden, a huge wave crashed down right on top of me and swept me off the ship. I was suddenly plunged into the bone-chilling water in the dark. Water filled my mouth and seemed to fill every part of my body. I doubted anyone had heard my cries. All around me was total darkness. I felt my body sinking down in the valley of the huge wave. I could not see the ship anywhere. For the first time, I realized what small, puny little beings we are to Mother Nature. I silently said my prayers and good-byes. I ceased my struggles and gave up all hope. Then suddenly, a huge wave lifted me up and deposited me right back on the deck of the ship. My knees buckled as I tried to stand up, so I crawled back to safety. All of that had happened in less than a minute. I had died and been reborn in a single moment. After that, I lived each day as a gift from heaven." Mr. Chang gathered our empty dishes and went back to the kitchen. He walked with lightness, between life and death.

"Well, that is the Tao, the force of nature. What takes away life will also give life. If the earth causes you to fall down, it also helps you to get up. Now, who is paying for this meal?" Sifu laughed as he watched us sitting there stone still.

"Allow me!" I said, rushing to grab the bill.

On the way out, as I walked on the pavement, I suddenly realized what our teacher had shown us. It was a lesson on the nature of spleen, earth force. What takes away will also give back. With each step, I felt Mother Earth tugging gently at my feet and then throwing them back: the ground that I walk on is alive, coiled with a deep spring. Since that day at the Dumpling House, even standing still, I can sense the skull-tingling force of Gaia, the living consciousness of earth.

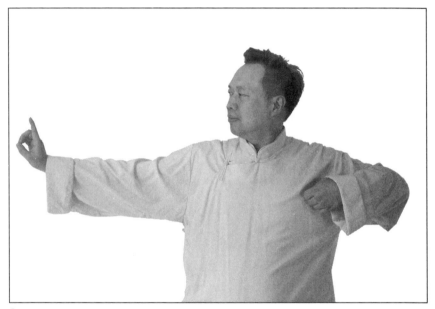

Lung

7

LUNGS: THE KNIGHTS IN SHINING ARMOR

*Translucent morning glory opens
Like a white parasol,
Shades iridescent bluebottle fly.*

IN TCM THEORY, within our body, each organ possesses its own unique consciousness. The consciousness of the lung has the spirit of protection and the emotion of grief. The lungs are the protectors of our internal organs. Their physical structure spreads out like an umbrella, shielding all other organs. Our lungs are the first barrier of defense between our internal environment and the outer world. They are also the first organ that gets attacked by external viruses and bacteria. In TCM, the lung is the organ from which energy flow originates; it is also the organ that functions with our very first breath. The lungs are called the *taiyin*, Supreme Yin, organ, or the organ that has the greatest space. If the surface area of the lungs were spread out, it would cover a handball court.

The best way to grasp the overall function of the lung is through the alchemical ritual of making hot cocoa. To review, in the alchemical ritual, we recreate a paradigm of our inner body, in which the different containers represent our internal organs, and the liquids we pour from one to another represent the fluids circulating between the different organs. The functions of the lung are symbolized in the fifth step of making hot cocoa, in the pouring of milk from a metal bowl into the hot cocoa mixture. The milk, the metal bowl, and the pouring of the mixture embody the three major aspects of the lungs' function.

The first aspect is their function of enriching and cooling, symbolized by the milk stored in the metal bowl. The lungs enrich the blood with oxygen and qi, and at the same time they cool the body, because the external oxygenated gas that they bring in is much cooler than the internal gas (mostly carbon dioxide) that they breathe out. Thus, in TCM, the freshly oxygenated blood in the arteries is cooler than the exhausted blood in the veins. For the venous blood also functions as a fluid heat sink by exchanging heat from cellular metabolic combustion. A weakening of the lung's coolant function will cause the body to become easily overheated.

A further aspect of this function of the lungs is that they direct the flow of qi. In TCM theory, it is the lung qi that is ultimately responsible for the enrichment and cooling of the blood, because it is the active force that moves the blood through the body. This relationship between qi and blood indicates the close relationship between the lungs and the heart. A lack of lung qi will result in stagnation of the blood circulation, and when the lung qi is deficient, there is not enough force to propel the blood, so the heart has to overwork in order to send the blood around the body. Without the cooling function of the lungs, the heart will become overheated, and the cardiac muscles can become damaged.

Work in a high-stress job or a sudden burst of high-impact activity will stress the heart and overheat it. According to TCM theory, excessive physical exercise, especially if done incorrectly, causes the heart to overheat and can actually damage the heart muscles. In the case of "weekend warriors" and their Saturday afternoon marathon jog, running is wonderful if you are conditioned, but if your lungs do not have the capacity to breathe fully, the heart becomes overheated. When the lungs are weakened and cannot breathe in enough oxygen or qi, the heart has to beat faster to compensate for the lack of qi. Similarly, in making hot chocolate, the milk is crucial, because it enriches and cools the hot cocoa to make it drinkable.

The second aspect of the lungs is their protective function, or immune response. In our alchemical ritual, this is represented by the metallic bowl, which contains the cooling milk. The metal symbolizes the lungs' function as guardian and protector against infection and the invasion of environmental pathogens. In the TCM model, the lungs are represented as an umbrella that shields all the organs beneath it. In TCM theory, the lungs generate the immune qi, or the defensive qi, and circulate it on the exterior of the body, the skin. This protective qi serves to fight and destroy infections, which is one of the major properties of the skin. The skin is the organ with which most external pathogens come into contact first; it is the first barrier between you and the environment. So, the lungs and skin are very closely related. Both are actively engaged in the interaction between the outer environment and our inner environment. The skin is our external barrier and the lungs are our internal barriers between the outer world and the inner world of our cells. Inside the lobes of the lung tissues, besides the rich network of blood capillaries, there is also a dense web of lymph vessels. They become the sentinels against foreign invaders from the air. Therefore, when smokers damage their lungs by inhaling noxious gases and carcinogenic particles, they deal a double blow to both their ability to breathe and the lungs' immune response.

When the lungs are healthy, there's a shine to the skin. When they are are unhealthy, the skin has a pale, ashen, grayish hue. In TCM, many skin diseases are attributed to weakness of the lungs and their functions. If you work or live in an enclosed environment without adequate ventilation, this will quickly affect your lungs. Observe office workers who work in small cubicles all day without any fresh air. When they emerge at the end of the day, their skin is ashen and parched. By contrast, look at farmers or apple pickers selling produce at the local farmers market—they always look like their skin is bursting with qi, and there's a shine to it. It's really amazing. And it will happen to you, too. If you spend a week in the country air, you will notice an improvement in your skin, not just because the air is good for your skin but because the air is also good for the lungs.

Invigorating the skin will help your breathing. An example of this is a TCM technique used to heal lung problems, called *gwa sa*, which means "scraping sand." A Chinese healer uses a smooth ceramic spoon, puts oil on the patient's back and chest, and scrapes vigorously, until the skin is almost bruised. Scraping the skin this way can relieve lung problems such as asthma or chronic coughs. This treatment is often used for Chinese children who have difficulty breathing. When I was a child, my mother did gwa sa to me with a silver coin, and it worked. This traditional Chinese method of healing should be done only by a trained healer, so please do not try this on your own. However, what you can do is use a good natural-bristle hairbrush to brush your whole body. This can help to invigorate your lungs. Also, I do not recommend wearing clothes made from synthetic fabrics, which prevent the free flow of air to your skin. Wear all natural fibers. The inflow of air can improve the health of your skin, lungs, and breathing.

The third function of the lungs is to generate a downward-directing force, symbolized in our alchemical ritual by the pouring of the mixture. What is this for? Why is it important? One of the main purposes of this downward force of the lung is the elimination of wastes. If the lungs are weak because of infection or some other condition, the downward force becomes too weak to push out the waste from the large intestine and colon. This results in constipation and the buildup of toxicity in the body. In TCM, constipation can be caused by weakness of the lung's downward function. In order to relieve chronic constipation, many TCM doctors will prescribe herbs to strengthen the lungs, as the constipation will be eliminated when the lungs become strong. I have observed that many patients who suffer from chronic constipation show weakness in their lung function and shallow breathing. A person who is constipated most likely will not be breathing too deeply. Of course, not everyone with shallow breathing has constipation. The old and the very young often become chronically constipated, because their lungs are naturally weak.

Weakness of the downward-directing force of the lungs can also explain the symptoms of coughing and shortness of breath. In both cases, the downward force is being counteracted by the upward force of the sickness. Observe that both in asthma and in coughing, there is a shallow upward expulsion of air.

Working with this downward force is central to the practice of the xi Healing Sound. To understand why this is so, think about how the xi sound is primarily a hissing sound. If you are a performing artist, you know the power of a hiss—all you need is a few people in the audience doing it: one in the left corner, one in the back, one in the front, and it will bring the curtain down! So the hissing sound of xi is a primal way of bringing energy downward, and this helps the downward direction of the lung's force.

The ancient Taoist masters were also aware that the xi sound was the sound for autumn. It is the sound of falling energy, falling leaves. In the woods during the autumn, if you keep quiet, you will hear a "hsss, hsss," which is the sound of leaves falling onto the ground, and a soft melancholy infiltrates your spirit. Perhaps that's why autumn is called fall.

So the lung likes things to go down, and the Healing Sound of the lung is to enhance this downward function. It is because of the lung's downward energy that in all Qigong breathing, practitioners are encouraged to breathe down to the soles of their feet. Thus the breathing is in harmony with the downward-directing flow of the lung's qi. On the other hand, if for some strange reason, you want to create an anti-Qigong practice, just instruct a student to breathe up into his head. You could call this some kind of "dark Qigong," because I'll wager that such a practitioner would eventually get sick.

Always practice with a deep, long breath. In this way, the Qigong breath enhances the lungs' natural downward flow and allows them to stay free of debris and infection. When the lungs are clear, their enriching and cooling functions can work properly to supply us with rich, cool, oxygenated blood.

May your breath be so deep that it penetrates to the core of
    the earth.

Long breath, long life!

General Healing Sounds Meditation

Practice the general Healing Sounds meditation as described on
pages 48–49. In preparing for the lung meditation, you will want to
pay special attention to the following:

- When you rest your hands on your knees with the palms down
  (or with your hands on your thighs with the palms up, if you
  find this more comfortable), stretch your thumbs slightly. The
  thumbs are the end points of the lung meridians and control the
  opening and closing of the lungs. Spreading your thumbs helps
  the lungs to open.

Lung Meditation: Taiyin Full Moon

Sit comfortably on a chair with your feet planted firmly on the floor
and your eyes gently closed but not shut tight. Let your palms rest
on your knees. Imagine that it is the middle of the night and there is
a full moon. As you breathe quietly, envision your lungs as inflatable
air chambers. The right lung contains three air chambers and the left
lung is composed of two. Imagine that each of these chambers has
its own ducts circulating the flow of air.

Imagine being in a vast open space filled with the clear light of
the full moon. Breathe in and visualize the moonlight streaming
through your right nostril down into the uppermost chamber of
your right lung. Let the whole right side of your chest inflate, and
then very softly turn your neck to the right, with the head just nod-
ding side to side. This allows you to further relax the right air duct.
Then, when you have done this, very simply say "How do you do?"
to your right lung.

Continue to breathe in the moonlight and allow the moonlight to stream down into the second air chamber on the right side. This time, just beneath the nipple, feel the movement, the sense of spaciousness, and allow the ribs to expand, and continue relaxing the right side of your neck. Finally, breathe in deeply and let the moonlight fill the lowest lobe of your right lung.

As all three lobes of your right lung are filled with light, be aware of the expansion and freedom in the whole right side of your body. It almost feels as if it is floating freely. Feel a sense of coolness on the right side, from the right nostril through the neck, and all the way to the lung. If you feel a slight lightheadedness, do not be afraid. Just pause gently. It is natural in most cases, as the brain is being filled with much more oxygen than it may be used to.

Now look within yourself and notice the difference between the right and left sides of your body. Be aware of the kinesthetic sensation of your respiration. Do you feel that your right side is freer and the air goes in more smoothly? Just having the awareness in your respiration will allow the breath to be more open and free.

Now let's balance the other side. Still sitting in the full moonlight, let the moonlight stream into the topmost air chamber of your left lung. Visualize the light entering through your nose, into the left top chamber of the lung, filling the upper lobe of the lung with silver moonlight. Now remember, the left lung has only two lobes, so continue breathing softly, inhaling deeper into the lowest lobe of the left lung, and let the light filter in. As you do so, relax the left side of your neck, again turning your head gently from side to side to facilitate relaxation of the neck muscles. You might be aware of a soft wet sensation, like a mist descending from the heavens into your head. As the mist condenses, the dewdrops from heaven start to drip down from the head to your heart. Can you almost hear the drip, drip, drip? From the heart, let these dewdrops expand to your whole lung, bringing healing energy there. Continue to allow your breath to become deeper and freer. Again, envision the mist descending from the heavens, this time allowing it to be illuminated, to become a rainbow. As this rainbow slowly descends from your head to your shoulders, feel a warm, ticklish sensation running across the whole breadth of your shoulders, down your upper and then lower arms until you feel little droplets of condensation trickling out your fingertips. Let all the darkness, grief, despair, and tension drip away.

To finish, very gently blow out a few times with your mouth, dispelling the pool of little dark droplets around you, and very gently say XI. Sense how the darkness and the despair disperse like fog and are absorbed by the environment around you. XI is a very soothing, sandy sound, like the breeze blowing through sand dunes and the sand rustling against the seaweed on the grass. By now, the air and surrounding environment are clear of despair and are filled with the clear light of a full-moon night.

Slowly allow your eyes to open, smile to yourself, smile to your lungs, and say "Hello, how do you do?" And one of these days, you might be surprised that you get a response from your lungs.

Very gently open your arms and stretch them up to the heavens, breathe in, and exhale saying "Ahh," and let your arms drop to your thighs. Do this three times, and on the last time shake your fingers, as if saying "I am feeling the force, I am feeling the force" or "I believe in Peter Pan," and then let them drop.

Lung Healing Sound Instruction: XI

Sound Component	Description
Consonant: X	X functions to cool the lungs. The consonant is like hissing steam from a teakettle.
Vowel: I	The *i* vowel sounds like *zeee*. The resulting humming resembles the buzzing of a honeybee.
Subvocal wind sound: *Hsss*	*Hsss* is a breathy nonvocal sound like the soft sigh of a cricket. There is a trailing-off of the XI sound as you come to the end of your breath.

Breath Integrals	Specifics
Tongue	The tip of the tongue should be held lightly between the teeth.
Mouth shape	Lips gently stretch to the side and expose the teeth.

Lung Healing Sound Vocal Instruction

In the Healing Sound XI, it is important to keep the eight breath integrals in a state of natural relaxation—especially the diaphragm, which you may recall is like a rubber band. During inhalation it stretches down and allows the lungs to expand. Then when we exhale, it snaps back up like a rubber band, and as it releases it floats way up under the ribs and pushes the air out from the lungs. The most important aspect of a full exhalation is that it allows the diaphragm to push out as much of the stagnant air as possible from the lungs' air sacs. Also remember the tongue position—you should place the tip of the tongue between your teeth, but do not bite it. Finally, pull back the lips as if you are hissing, and make sure your throat and larynx remain relaxed and open (see fig. 7.1). There are three components to the Healing Sound XI:

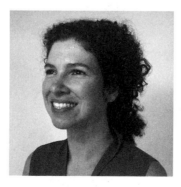

FIGURE 7.1. *XI*

- There is the consonant *x*, which sounds like a hissing teakettle. This helps to release the excessive buildup of heat.
- There is the vowel sound of *i*, which is done very nasally and actually sounds more like *zeee*. This helps to strengthen the organ of the lung.
- Finally, there is the subvocal wind sound, which is a silent hissing sound of *hsss*. It almost sounds like the hissing steam escaping from a teakettle. It is a very gentle hissing sound, done without any malice. This is to nourish the organ.

Practicing the Healing Sound is like making a three-layer sandwich. The top layer is the consonant, the middle part is the vowel, and the bottom layer is the wind sound. It is important to do all three aspects of the Healing Sound.

Try the xi sound now. Sit or stand comfortably. Allow the body to be soft, keeping the whole length of the torso relaxed, from your abdomen to your throat. Let the tip of your tongue touch between your teeth. As for the pitch, do what is natural. Women can do a higher pitch, and men can have a lower one. Repeat the sound three times.

Lung Healing Sound Movement Instruction: Drawing the Bow

The overall movement image of the Healing Sound for the lungs is that of drawing a bow and arrow.

- *Gather.* Stand with feet shoulder-width apart or sit on chair. Fold the hands overlapping at the Elixir Field, three inches below the navel (see fig. 7.2). Remember, Healing Sounds Qigong can be done either sitting down or standing, as you prefer.
- *Arise.* Inhale and softly curl your fingers into loose fists, and cross your arms. Slowly let your crossed arms rise up from the Elixir Field to the heart and stop at the chest, as if giving yourself a gentle hug (see figs. 7.3, 7.4, and 7.5) As the arms rise up

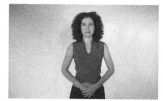

FIGURE 7.2. *Gather*

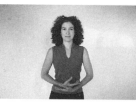

FIGURE 7.3. *Arise*

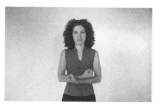

FIGURE 7.4

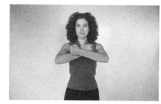

FIGURE 7.5

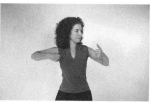

FIGURE 7.6. *Draw*

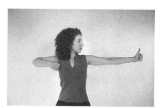

FIGURE 7.7

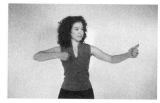

FIGURE 7.8. *Cross*

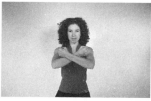

FIGURE 7.9

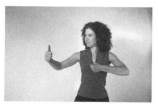

FIGURE 7.10. *Draw*

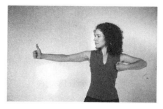

FIGURE 7.11

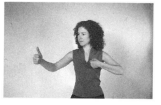

FIGURE 7.12. *Cross*

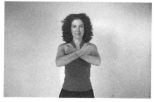

FIGURE 7.13

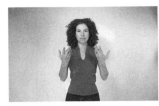

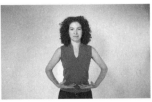

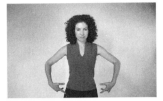

FIGURE 7.14. *Descend*   FIGURE 7.15   FIGURE 7.16. *Gather*

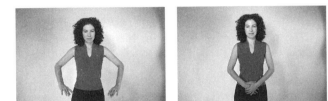

FIGURE 7.17   FIGURE 7.18

to the chest, feel the back open up and let more breath into the lungs. Feel how your chest rises and falls with your breath. The main point in most Qigong movement is to keep a soft, open, easy pose. The fists should be held loosely and not squeezed tight. Any unnecessary tension will impede the movement of your lungs.

- *Draw.* Exhale with the XI sound. Gently extend your left "bow" fist at shoulder level out to the side with the thumb pointing up. Simultaneously, turn your head to the left and focus your gaze on your thumb. Imagine that you are sighting a target to your left. At the same time, draw the right "arrow" fist to the right, located proximal to the armpit, as if you were drawing a bow; keep the elbow down (see figs. 7.6 and 7.7). Now maintain this Draw posture for the lungs. As you make the lung Healing Sound, XI, feel the vibration traveling down the whole length of your arms. In drawing the right fist, do not use force. Imagine that the bow-string is made of a strand of spider's silk, keep your fist loose, and let it rest on your chest.

- *Cross.* Inhale, relax your arms, then gather and cross them over the chest again (see figs. 7.8 and 7.9). Relax. Take a moment to feel your chest. Check whether your chest is soft and relaxed and not tight and tensed. Observe any difference in the movement of your breath. Be aware of whether your breathing seems smoother or deeper.
- *Draw.* Exhale with the XI sound. Gently extend your right "bow" fist at shoulder level out to the side with the thumb pointing up. Simultaneously, turn your head to the right and focus your gaze on your thumb. Imagine that you are sighting a target to your right. At the same time, draw the left "arrow" fist to the left, located proximal to the armpit, as if you were drawing a bow; keep the elbow down (see figs. 7.10 and 7.11). Maintain the posture in a relaxed manner. Allow the vibration of the Healing Sound to travel up the whole length of your arm into your lungs.
- *Repeat.* Repeat the steps of Draw, Cross, Draw to the left and right, up to three times.
- *Cross.* Finally, gently bring your arms together and cross them over your chest once more (see figs. 7.12 and 7.13). Breathe naturally, relax, and notice any difference in the physical movement of your breathing. Has it become easier? Has it become deeper?
- *Descend.* To finish, slowly unfurl your fists and spread your arms as if you were parting a curtain. Lower your hands very gently to your abdomen (see figs. 7.14 and 7.15).
- *Gather.* Inhale and unfurl the hands outward as if they were making a small rippling motion. Overlap the hands at the Elixir Field (see figs. 7.16, 7.17, and 7.18). If standing, gently shake your legs. If seated, let your spine shudder like a dog shaking off water. This releases any built-up strain or tension.

Refining the Lung Healing Sound Qigong

As in the preceding chapter, if you have shoulder problems, do not raise your arms to shoulder level. Modify the movement without straining your body. In turning your head to the side, make sure that you do not tilt your head back or strain your neck by twisting it too hard. I strongly advise beginning students to turn their heads only forty-five degrees to the corner, rather than to the side. This will reduce neck strain. Gazing to the side or diagonally to the corner has the effect of stretching the neck muscles and opening the carotid artery along the side of the neck, thus improving blood circulation to the head.

The Draw the Bow posture helps to support the lungs so that they breathe in more air. As you draw the bow, keep your back plumb erect without arching the lower back or shifting your weight to your heels.

Taoists see the cosmos in terms of numerological permutations. Performing three repetitions invokes the three realms: heaven, human, and earth. Although there is no harm in doing four or five repetitions, in the spirit of alchemy I have adhered to the classical schema of Taoist numerology.

Healing Sound Story: He Seemed to Move a Bit Stiffly

"His movements seemed a bit stiff" was a comment by one of the guests who saw Ben's Taiji demonstration at our school's annual Chinese New Year celebration.

"Stiff! Ben has no legs," I replied. The guest was wide-eyed and his mouth dropped open.

Ben was a Vietnam veteran whose legs were blown off below the knees by a mine explosion. He had come to me because of phantom pain and also wanted me to help him learn to walk more naturally with his prostheses.

"I have seen many doctors, and they all told me that the pain I feel is some sort of phantom pain," Ben told me. "Every time I walk with my prostheses I feel this sharp, cutting pain that shoots up from my toes to my knees. I know that I don't have toes anymore, but that is what it feels like to me."

I watched Ben walk. He put each foot down as if the floor were strewn with broken glass. It was obvious to an observer that he was wearing prostheses. I knew that I had to deal with his phantom pain before Ben could walk with a more natural gait.

I started by working with Ben on his breathing, which was very locked and arrested. He breathed with a laborious pulling-in of air as if he were drowning.

"Place your palms on your chest and feel the earth beneath you. Feel how solid it is, and melt yourself into the floor," I instructed Ben as he lay on the floor.

Suddenly, his body started to thrash wildly like a trout leaping out of the water.

"Sorry, that always happens when I start to relax," Ben apologized.

"That's fine. Do not repress the spontaneous release. Let it unwind itself slowly. But focus on your palms and feel how your breath is flowing," I continued.

His legs started to twitch. "My toes are really hurting me," Ben moaned.

I used my intuition to guide me to the energy field of his toes and started to gently massage the "phantom toes." I could feel a prickling sensation on my palms, and suddenly a searing heat was released. Being trained in the energetic field of Qigong, I was not surprised, although I was not touching anything but thin air. As I closed my eyes, I could imagine Ben's toes cramped in a spasm of pain. With my fingers, I gently massaged his toes' energy field.[1]

"Ah. The pain went away." Ben relaxed as the twitch gradually died off and he started to drift into the twilight zone of a wakeful-sleep state. His breath started to smooth out. With the acknowledgment and release of his phantom pain, Ben was also able to let go of his grief over the loss of his limbs. The emotion of grief hurts the function of the lungs. By releasing his grief, he was able to recover the natural full capacity of his lungs.

"Now, Ben, as you walk, imagine that your toes are spreading out and you can trust the ground." I led Ben through the slow dance of the Taiji movements. His face broke into a large grin as he felt the earth with his "toes."

After Ben and I had worked together for three years, he demonstrated the Taiji form at the New Year celebration. Afterward, I related the response of the guest to Ben that his form was a bit stiff.

"I'll take that as a compliment," Ben chuckled.

Since working with Ben, I have had more opportunities to work with other clients who had organs or parts of their body removed. As I work with their physical bodies, I always pay attention to balancing their missing "energetic" organ or body part as well.

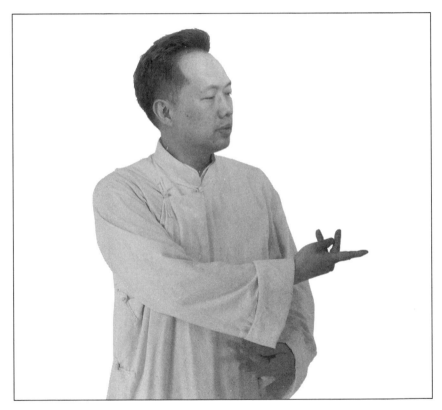

Kidney

KIDNEYS: FIRE AND WATER

Primordial water,
Dark and fertile within the reflection of the moon,
Water and fire dance the Creation of life.

THE KIDNEY is an unusual organ system. It is the only organ in the TCM system that has both water and fire characteristics. Whereas other organs have only one element (the heart is fire, warming; the lungs are metal, cooling), in the kidney, water and fire combine. When Chinese doctors speak of the kidney, they include the adrenal glands, which rest right on top of the kidneys. If you have ever eaten chicken kidneys, you may have noticed those little areas on top that look like pieces of fat. Those are the adrenal glands. The kidney actually is an organ with two different systems: the kidney itself, which is watery, and the adrenal gland on top, which is fiery.

According to TCM, the kidneys serve as the rechargeable batteries of your body. At birth they are given a full charge, and as you age, they start to degenerate. Even though you recharge them, there's only a certain amount that they can be recharged before they become useless. Similarly, in TCM, the kidney is endowed with a prenatal life force. When you are born, this force starts to degenerate, and when it is depleted, you have the effects of old age and eventually death. This is why Taoists and Qigong healers are fixated on the kidney. A well-known Chinese expression is *ji san*, which you say when someone treasures life. Literally translated, *ji* is to know and *san* is kidney, so to treasure life is to know your kidneys, because they are the battery, the reservoir of life.

In TCM, all the essential fluids, including blood, sexual fluid, saliva, bone marrow, and cerebrospinal fluid, are generated and controlled by the kidney, which is like a reservoir, giving out streams to cultivate and nourish all the different fields of the body. For example, the blood, which nourishes every part of the body, flows out from the kidney reservoir to nourish the heart. Now it may seem a funny thing to think that the heart needs the nourishment of blood, but that's exactly why people have heart attacks: they don't have enough blood supply to the muscles of the heart, because their coronary arteries get blocked. Also from this reservoir, there is an outflow of what in TCM are called the seminal or ovarian fluids (which in modern medicine are called endocrine hormones) to nourish our reproductive organs.

For women, the kidneys play several roles. They are involved in the menstrual cycle, because they rule the cyclic flow of blood, and are therefore responsible for any menstrual sickness or disorder. When girls have their menarche, their kidneys blossom. The energy pops them open. When the kidneys blossom, the skin is very shiny and there's a lot of moisture, very much like a ripe, plump orange hanging on a tree, ready to be picked. As the kidney opens, a girl has her first menstruation. This is due to the kidney qi supplying it with sexual reproductive fluid. As a woman grows older, her kidneys start to run dry, and when she reaches the age of forty-nine (according to the *I Ching*), the kidney's reproductive fluid is exhausted and she goes through menopause. For men, this occurs at age fifty-six. His sexual potency, desire, and hormonal levels will begin to decline parallel to a woman's menopause.

The kidney is also responsible for producing and maintaining the health of bone marrow and cerebrospinal fluid (CSF). The bone marrow nourishes the bones and is also involved in producing blood. With regard to CSF, from the TCM point of view, the kidney has a direct channel to the brain (this is the basis of the hollow organ meditation on pages 126–28). Therefore, when the CSF (which in TCM is referred to as brain fluid) runs dry, you can become senile and develop diseases such as Parkinson's or Alzheimer's. We know now that the brain needs an adequate supply of so-called sex hormones such as testosterone and progesterone. When this runs dry, the brain starts to degenerate. That's the watery aspect of the kidney, which flows very slowly and gradually, moving like the tide, according to the lunar cycle.

Now for the other aspect of the kidney, its fiery aspect. First, the kidney is considered to be the origin of the triple heater, whose role is to heat up the three main parts of our body. Here is a little scenario to illustrate the fiery part of the kidney: Half a million years ago, early in the morning, a caveman stumbles out of his cave, still half asleep, to find himself a little breakfast. All of a sudden, out leaps a saber-toothed tiger. Instantly the caveman wakes up, jumps out of the way, gives a loud scream, and luckily escapes.

What allowed the caveman to change states so quickly is the kidney or, more specifically, the adrenal gland, which sits on top of the kidney. When it responds to a threat or to stress, it secretes adrenaline, and the response is immediate. That's the fiery aspect of the kidney, as fire is very fast acting. Because of this, the kidney is highly susceptible to immediate stress. You can see the effect of stress in the kidney right away. Unfortunately, once the kidney has been stressed, it takes quite a long time for the caveman to calm down—he's hyped up, ready to run or fight for his life.

In modern times, we use artificial stress to stimulate the kidney. For example, people who live in northern climates, where the winters are long and dark, drink many more cups of coffee a day than people living in the tropics. Some people drink twelve cups of coffee a day in order to stimulate themselves. When you constantly stimulate the kidney, you are turning its flame up very high. Outwardly, those people are nice and bright, vivacious, and talk a mile a minute.

And then what happens? They can spontaneously have chronic fatigue, go into deep depression, and do something like ride a motorcycle off a mountain trail. According to TCM, long-term stress without any respite can cause deep depression and even suicide.

Another fire function of the kidney is to monitor the body's metabolic rate. It turns the flame a little higher when you have more things to do. When you are young, your metabolic rate is higher so you can eat a lot of food and still stay skinny. But as you get older, your metabolic rate slows. The fire is not as strong, but you are throwing the same kind of fuel onto it. Then the flame becomes smoky, and therefore the metabolism can no longer digest the food totally, and it creates a lot of debris in the system. That's the problem with professional football players. Even after they stop playing football, they still eat like football players, but because their metabolic rate is no longer as high as it was when they were playing football, they gain a lot of weight.

How does stress affect the kidney? Here's a story: a high-level stockbroker works hard all day, and to relax after his stressful job he goes to a gym and does high-impact aerobics. According to TCM, this doesn't work, because it is burning the candle at both ends: he is actually stressing his body further. Then one day he doesn't want to move anymore and has a mental breakdown. In some experiments done on animals in which they are stressed repeatedly, sectioning their kidneys show that they have had internal hemorrhaging.

Therefore, reducing stress means not stressing your body further. If you want the kidneys to stay open and not be blocked, use the kidney Healing Sound CHU, which works by using very subtle vibrations to heal the organ. This is achieved by lightly touching the molars together when doing the Healing Sound because this vibrates the bones; and because the kidneys are responsible for bone growth, it cleanses the bone marrow as well as going down further to clear the kidney of any congestion.

According to the ancient Taoist masters, the way to health lies in the symbolism of water above and fire below. The special Healing Sound that they chose, CHU, expresses both the fire quality of the kidney (which is the *ch*, the hissing sound) and the watery sound of subterranean water (the gurgling *u*).

With each step you take, make sure that you walk with very deliberate awareness, so you do not spill the water of the kidney and put out the flame. And so too the reverse: do not live such a stimulated life that you turn the flame way up and burn the pot dry.

General Healing Sounds Meditation

Practice the general Healing Sounds meditation as described on pages 48–49. In preparing for the kidney meditation, you will want to pay special attention to the following:

- Since the kidneys' energy points are located at the hollows of your feet, sit with your legs spread to the width of your shoulders and curl your toes slightly as if you are sucking up water from the earth. This has the effect of drawing the fluid up from the feet back to the heart.
- Pay special attention to keeping your spine naturally erect, like an unstrung bow. In TCM diagnosis, a weak back is a sign of poor kidney function. Thus, strengthening the back indirectly helps to restore the health of the kidneys. Initially, you may find that your back becomes fatigued quite quickly, but with perseverance and practice, the spinal muscles will be strengthened. Then you can sit at ease even for a long period of time.

Kidney Healing Sound Meditation

I have included two kidney meditations because the kidney functions in a dual way, as the organ of watery coolness and as a fiery adrenaline high. Taoist practitioners have long noticed that a special kind of fire exists within the kidney. From modern science, we know that the adrenal glands are located above the kidneys; their function helps us to keep alert and ready for danger.

Try both meditations and feel for yourself which one seems

better for you. Without a face-to-face diagnosis, I cannot tell which one is better for any one person. Both kidney meditations can have profound effects on the organs and will do no harm. It is just that you may find one more fitting for you than the other.

KIDNEY MEDITATION 1: HOLLOWNESS

The usefulness of a bowl is in its hollowness;
The usefulness in a room is in its spaciousness.

—*Tao Te Ching*

Sit comfortably. Let your feet rest firmly on the ground. If you are sitting on a chair, let your palms rest on your knees, let your eyes close, roll the tip of your tongue so it touches the upper palate, and just take a few moments to breathe in and breathe out. Move your body to notice any area where you feel there is tension, and release the tension.

Now, envision your kidneys. Visualize them as two lumps of clay located in your middle back. Be aware of the shape and the texture of the kidney. Some people will experience it as very dry, and others as very wet. Visualize using your hand to gently knead the clay of the kidney, breathing in and breathing out. If it is too dry, swallow, and as you swallow, bring some of the saliva into the kidney and moisten the clay—the lump of clay that is your kidney—and knead it until it is nice and soft, as if you were making pottery.

Now, very gently with your energized hands, from both sides of the kidneys, stretch a long piece of clay from each one down toward your navel. Slowly, without breaking the pieces as you stretch them out, breathe into them and allow them to become hollow: two hollow tubes, one from the left kidney, one from the right kidney. Bring them down and allow them to meet and join as one at the area of your navel. Then, as the tube continues further down, let it diverge into two and go into your gonads. For women, let it divert and extend into the area of your ovaries, and for men, let it continue to descend until reaching your testicles. Now allow the ends of the tubes to become attached to the ovaries or the testes. Then, breathe into them, so that they become two hollow spheres. Now fill them with light. Fill them with fluid. Fill them with jing, your procreative essence. And take a moment to pause there.

Now work backward and retrace the paths, going from the hollow spheres of the gonads, up through the tubes, left and right emerging at the navel, going up, and then diverting back to the left and right kidneys. Then, from the kidneys I would like you to shape and form another two tubes. This time the tubes from the left and the right go up and merge at the heart. Then from the heart they continue as a single tube, going up the back of your throat, through your neck and reaching all the way up into your brain, to the level of your eyebrows. At the end of this tube, breathe and slowly let it billow out into a sphere about the size of a walnut. Now breathe and fill the hollow of the whole structure, the whole endocrine structure. Fill the hollow with soft fluids.

Finally, fill the space of the five hollows: the central brain hollow, the kidney hollows, and then your gonad hollows. As you breathe, synchronize the movement of the brain, kidneys, and gonads. Feel them expanding and contracting with the breath, as if they were one single organism with a life of its own. Fundamentally, all those organs are not solid. They are filled with space. When the organ becomes solid, that is when you have problems. You want to keep a sense of spaciousness in the hollow endocrine system.

To finish, inhale and open your arms and spread your hands out to the side, blossoming out from the heart. Go back to that hollow of the endocrine system, feeling the whole hollow expanding, filling with light and moisture and golden fluid, and smile to your kidneys. Sometimes the kidneys may not smile back and are actually grouchy. Sometimes the kidneys act like a cat. That's all right—continue smiling. And very gently, turn your palms down and let them rest on your knees.

Slowly come back. Sense how you feel inside. Feel a sense of spaciousness. Take a deep inhalation and slowly let your eyes open. As they open, stretch your hands up to the heavens. Then drop them very fast into your lap and exhale. Inhale and stretch your hands out to the sides. Exhale and let them drop. Finally, inhale and stretch your hands behind your chair, turning left and right. Slowly bring your hands back to the front, and exhale.

KIDNEY MEDITATION 2: LUNAR AMBER

Primordial water,
Dark and fertile within the reflection of the moon,
Water and fire, the lunar cyclic flow of tides.

Imagine sitting on the beach of a calm lake, the primordial lake, hearing the sound of waves, letting the mind follow the sound of waves coming and going. Allow your breath to synchronize with the flow of the tide. The full moonlight with its gentle soothing touch descends like a luminous liquid stream into the middle of your brain. Allow the lunar nectar to condense into a single drop of amber right behind your third eye, the space between your eyebrows.

With an almost audible plop, the luminous amber drops down into your kidneys. Visualize your kidneys as a shiny black translucence, like obsidian. As the amber drops into the kidneys, you may feel a sudden release and simultaneously a drawing-in of the kidney. Visualize the amber light spreading outward from the kidneys, illuminating the darkness of the kidney with light.

Let this light stream down further into your sex organs. Feel the connection between the brain, the kidneys, and the sex organs connected by the filament of light. Breathe gently to enhance this filament of light.

Now, continue to extend this light filament down to the soles of your feet. Feel a soft warmth at the bottom of your feet. Allow this warmth to rise up like mist and bathe your whole body in light.

Kidney Healing Sound Instruction: CHU

Sound Component	Description
Consonant: *Ch*	*Ch* functions to release stress/heat from the kidneys.
Vowel: *U*	The *u* vowel sound combined with the above consonant is like the sound of a "choo-choo" train.
Subvocal wind sound: *Sch*	*Sch* is a breathy nonvocal sound, like the soft sigh of the wind. There is a trailing-off of the CHU sound as you come to the end of your breath.

Breath Integrals	Specifics
Tongue	The tip rolls and curls back slightly toward the back of the mouth.
Teeth	Molars touch gently as if holding a soft piece of chewing gum. The teeth should vibrate during the Healing Sound.
Mouth shape	Lips are slightly pursed and rounded.

Kidney Healing Sound Vocal Instruction

Before we do the kidney Healing Sound, let's start with our Himalayan AH breath. What do we use as an image for the kidneys? Imagine that you are walking down a very cold street, the wind is blowing your hair, and you're all covered up, looking like an Egyptian mummy. When you finally arrive at your destination, you open the door and it is warm, and you see three little girls all saying hi to you. You take off your coat and your muffler and you say AH. Repeat the AH. Really let it out, feeling the joyousness of those three little girls greeting you. Do it one last time. Those three little girls represent your mind, your body, and your speech.

When you do the Healing Sound CHU, the sound is composed of three parts: The first is the consonant, the firm *ch*. The consonant's function is to release excessive heat and, in the case of the kidney, stress.

The second part of the Healing Sound CHU is a vowel, *u*. To make this sound properly, you have to very gently bite down with your molars, imagining that you have a very thin piece of gold foil that you just barely indent with the molars, not breaking it. Or, pretend that you are holding a thin piece of chewing gum between your molars and go *u*. Roll your tongue back as you say that *u*. It's a kind of guttural growling and serves to strengthen the kidneys.

Finally, the third part of the Healing Sound is the subvocal wind sound, which is very breathy. This sound is like a *sch*. It's almost inaudible, which is why it is called subvocal. Never attend a subvocal choir performance, because you will not hear anything! When you're subvocalizing, you are opening your windpipe. This is very relaxing and comfortable, and it nourishes the organ.

Now practice the sound. Without clenching your teeth, touch your molars together very gently so you can vibrate your teeth. As for the tongue, let the tip of it roll back as far as it can (see fig. 8.1). Now, gently say CHU. In general, for women it is a higher pitch and

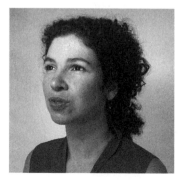

FIGURE 8.1. *CHU*

for men it is a lower one. Find a pitch that you are comfortable with. When you get the right pitch, you feel a vibration all over your jaw. The point is to vibrate the bone. Do it again, and this time you can slightly round your middle back so you can vibrate the kidney.

Kidney Healing Sound Movement Instruction

- *Gather.* Overlap the palms at the Elixir Field, three finger-widths below the navel. Women should place their right palm closest to their body. Men should place their left palm closest to their body (see fig. 8.2).
- *Open.* Inhale, opening the palms like orchid petals. Unfurl them inward so that the backs of the palms almost touch (see fig. 8.3).
- *Blossom.* Continue to inhale. Gather the tips of the thumb, the middle finger, and the ring finger of each hand, and extend the index finger and pinkie. This forms the orchid mudra (see fig. 8.4). Continue to curl the hands inward, until the palms are facing upward (see fig. 8.5). Join the hands together like two blossoms from a single sprig.

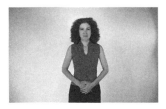

FIGURE 8.2. *Gather*

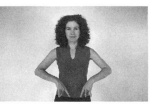

FIGURE 8.3. *Open*

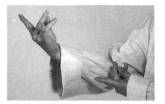

FIGURE 8.4. *Orchid Mudra*

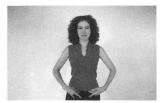

FIGURE 8.5. *Blossom*

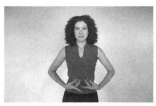

FIGURE 8.6. *Arise*

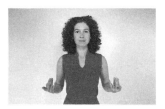

FIGURE 8.7. *Swirl Out*

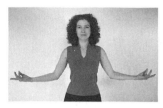

FIGURE 8.8

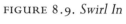

FIGURE 8.9. *Swirl In*

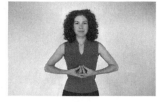

FIGURE 8.10

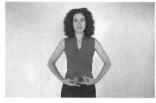

FIGURE 8.11. *Descend*

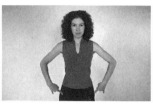

FIGURE 8.12. *Gather*

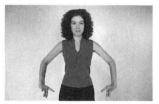

FIGURE 8.13

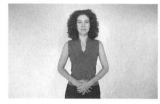

FIGURE 8.14

- *Arise.* Keep inhaling, raise the hands to just beneath the ribs, and slightly round your lower back as if you are bending down to smell the flower (see fig. 8.6).
- *Swirl Out.* Exhale with the CHU sound and swipe the hands in an arc about forty-five degrees in front of the body, keeping the elbows in (see figs. 8.7 and 8.8). Keep the movement synchronized with the full exhalation of the Healing Sound. As the hands swirl out, the exhalation is completed.
- *Swirl In.* Inhale fully, and gather the hands back to the region just beneath the ribs (see figs. 8.9 and 8.10). Repeat the Swirl Out and Swirl In phases three to six times.

- *Descend.* Exhale, and let the hands slowly drop down to the abdomen, maintaining the orchid mudra (see fig. 8.11).
- *Gather.* Inhale, and release the mudra by opening the fingers. Unfurl the hands outward so that they trace a small semicircle in the air. Overlap the hands at the Elixir Field (see figs. 8.12, 8.13, and 8.14).

Refining the Kidney Healing Sound Qigong

In the orchid mudra, the fingers become the orchid's central pistils, stigma, and outer petals. This mudra has subtle effects in stimulating and balancing the endocrine and reproductive glands, as the pistils and stigma are the flower's sexual and reproductive organs, emitting nectars and fragrances, their sexual pheromones. Sometimes you may even smell a sweet scent while doing the Qigong.

In the Swirl In and Swirl Out movement phases, the hands move lightly like wind-blown blossoms swaying. As you move, envision your hands as a sprig of purple blossoms in the morning light, dancing gently to the soft zephyr. Droplets of pure nectar drip from the fingertips.

Healing Sound Story: The Wanderer

"Hi, this is Bo. I am back and I would like to visit." My answering machine replayed the message.

Bo began his studies with me six years ago. After completing a year of studies in Qigong, he began his "Wandering Project" as a photojournalist and explorer traveling to distant parts of the world. He remains one of my long-distance students.

When he began studying with me, Bo was a young man in his early twenties. He had long blond hair and a thin wispy cloud of golden beard. He came to study the Healing Sounds and Qigong because of a special condition. After a group class, Bo stayed behind to ask me a question.

"I fainted in the bathroom and my girlfriend had to drag me to the bed," was how Bo explained his initial complaint.

"How many times did this occur? And do you remember what circumstances accompanied your fainting?" I was trying to be tactful in ascertaining whether Bo had taken any psychotropic drugs.

"Well, I fainted twice in the last three months. The first time happened after making love. Afterward I went to the bathroom, and while I was urinating I just fainted. The second time was a couple of months later and the same thing happened." He was a little embarrassed.

I asked Bo whether he had seen a doctor. He replied that he had and that they could not find anything unusual in his blood work. The doctor just told him to take it easy.

"This is actually a common occurrence in some men," I told him. "In Chinese medicine, sexual activity is related to the kidneys. After you made love, your kidney essence was temporarily depleted. When you tried to urinate, all the blood was drained from your brain to flow down to the kidneys as you relaxed your urinary tract and your kidneys. At that moment, due to the lack of blood, you blacked out. There are a couple of simple solutions to your dilemma. The obvious one is not to have any more sex."

Rolling his eyes, he asked, "What is the other option?"

"Well, an ancient Taoist practice is to clench your teeth gently as you urinate. This will prevent the essence of the kidneys from being depleted along with the urine. Try to keep inhaling at the same time. It will be difficult in the beginning but you will get used to it. By the way, as you inhale, try to silently make the sound CHU, I replied.

Bo seemed a little perplexed, but he practiced the method diligently every time he urinated. He found it difficult to urinate and inhale while clenching his teeth at the same time, but after a day or so, he was able to do it.[1]

After a year, the fainting never occurred again. Then Bo decided to leave his job as assistant in a photography studio and to roam the earth. As the qi of his kidneys was restored, Bo was able to make profound life decisions, an expression of healthy kidneys. Midlife crisis is due to the sexual energy changing in a man's kidneys, and this provokes him to look at his life with critical eyes. For Bo, this occurred in his twenties.

He left his Swedish model girlfriend and moved to the Himalayas to photograph the elements of earth and air. After three years, he came back to visit me and shared with me the exhilaration of solitary life in the foothills of the Himalayas in Nepal. His photographs of the blue sky and clouds as well as the dry animal bones of the Himalayas were breathtaking. The photographs inspired me to create the Himalayan AH breath for my Healing Sounds seminars.

The next three years Bo spent living in a coastal town in Ireland, photographing the ocean. This sojourn was for his next element, water. Again he came back and shared with me news of his latest project. This time, there were many stories of romance and songs. The photographs of the Irish coast seemed to express the eternal battle between land and ocean—each wanted to reclaim what it had lost.

"So where are you going for your fire project?" I handed Bo a cup of tea.

"Well, in Ireland, I met an Australian woman. She invited me to trek across the Australian outback. I am going to join her in a few days," Bo replied.

"Well, watch out! I think that the fire woman may get you stuck in the outback." I laughed.

I expect another call from Bo three years from now, as he explores the fire element—or maybe when he sends me an invitation to his wedding in Australia.

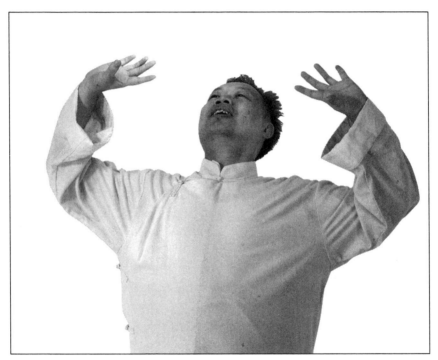

Triple Heater

9

TRIPLE HEATER:
THE ORGANIC FURNACE

Three crazy Taoists laugh so hard
They fall down on their backs.
"Why?" you ask.
"Don't you know laughter is the best medicine for old age?"
*   as they point to the moon.*

O UNDERSTAND the triple heater's functions, we
can use the analogy of an old loft building with three floors.
The triple heater, in this model, serves as both the structural
elements that separate each floor as well as the hot water heater and
radiator system that links the three floors together. Hence, one of
the triple heater's major functions is to distribute and regulate heat
in the building. Plus, sometimes one can use the radiator to com-
municate with the neighbors—for example, when they play loud
heavy-metal music. If one gently taps the radiator with a stick, the
sound will travel to the next floor. Thus, the triple heater also serves
as a means of communication between the three floors.

What are the three floors? The top floor corresponds to the
upper heater, which serves as the heating and communication agent
for the lungs and heart—the cardiopulmonary system. The second
floor corresponds to the middle heater, which serves as the heating

and communication agent for the digestive system of the spleen and stomach. The ground floor represents the lower heater, which serves as the heating and communication agent for the kidneys, liver, and reproductive organs. Running throughout the three floors are the ducts and meridians, energy pathways that connect the three heaters. The ducts and meridians must remain in a state of openness for the triple heater to function properly. Any blockage in the connective agents will result in a weakened immune response.

In an old building, sometimes in the middle of winter, the hot water cannot reach the top floor—the first two floors are nice and hot, but the third floor is usually cold. Similarly, when energy of the triple heater is insufficient to reach the top floor, one has cold hands and feet. The triple heater's energy is not strong enough to carry the heat from the core of the body to the periphery of the fingers and toes. Therefore, the name "triple heater" is appropriate—it is a means of warming your body. Health is warm and soft; sickness is cold and stiff.

Of course, if the radiators are overactive, then one's body becomes overly hot. It is as if the boiler in the basement is ready to explode, so you need to run downstairs and quickly let out the steam. Similarly, when one is excessively hot, either from overactivity, sickness, stress, or taking psychotropic drugs, one's body, hands, and feet become sweaty and overly hot. This is the result of an overactive, overstimulated triple heater. The Healing Sound of HEY serves as a way of letting out this steam. Of course, if the excessive heat is due to a medical condition, you must seek medical help as well.

In TCM, triple heater diagnosis employs the simple analogy of radiators in a building. If the radiator on the top floor starts to leak, it drips down to the second floor. In other words, if the respiratory system (the top floor) has an infection that's not taken care of, the infected phlegm will leak down to the second floor, the digestive system, which will become bloated and blocked.

What happens if the infection of the digestive system cannot be stopped? Then, just like a leak that is not fixed, the disease will continue down to the next floor. Now the people on the first floor say, "Oh, look, there's a leak in our ceiling." By the time the infection from the top floor has leaked all the way down to the bottom floor (the kidneys and liver), the disease has developed to an extremely serious stage. The kidneys and liver are two of our most essential and vulnerable organs. This is the end stage of a grave infection, and usually by now the patient shows signs of serious weakness.

Here is the progress of the infection in terms of the three elements of the triple heater. When the infection occurs at the upper heater, one might have a relatively high temperature. Then, when the sickness degenerates to the middle heater at the digestive system, the body temperature becomes even higher, reaching its peak fever. But when the infection crashes down to the last floor, extending deeper into the kidneys and the liver, the temperature actually drops. This dropping of the body temperature is a dangerous sign. The body is "burned up" and has depleted its immune energy. There is nothing left to fight the infection.

In milder cases, when a low-grade infection reaches and stays at the kidneys and liver, you can have chronic fatigue syndrome. The patient is tired all the time. There may also be acute flare-ups, but the flare-ups are usually not hot enough to elicit an immune response that can get rid of the infection. Therefore, according to TCM, chronic fatigue is a syndrome in which the infection has moved through the three heaters from top to bottom. The immune system is not strong enough to eradicate the infection, and therefore patients with chronic fatigue syndrome continue to have low-grade fever and abnormal body temperature fluctuations.

Using this diagnostic principle, if a patient consults a Chinese doctor complaining of symptoms associated with a urinary-tract infection, the doctor may ask if the patient has had any respiratory problems in the past several months (usually the answer is yes). The next question is whether the patient has taken care of it appropriately (usually the answer is no) and finally, how his or her digestion has been in the last few months (usually not so good). Then the Chinese doctor will see that the infection has moved downward from the respiratory system through the digestive system and now is in the urinary system.

So, going back to our building model, what does a good plumber do when there is a leak on the bottom floor? A master plumber does not simply patch the ceiling as if that were the actual source of the leakage. Rather, he will first mop up the wetness—in the case of the urinary tract infection, this would mean curing that infection. Furthermore, he will go to the top floor, the upper heater, to investigate and plug up the real source of the leakage. Hence, a good Chinese doctor might give the patient a dual prescription of herbs to heal both the lower and upper heaters, the urinary and respiratory systems. In contrast, if the patient receives only repeated doses of antibiotics to treat the urinary infection, the infection may clear up, but it will recur. Remember that in treating any sickness, the three "floors" of the triple heater must be taken into account. Treating just the symptoms of an infection or illness will provide only temporary relief. Hence, the sublime curative effects of TCM and Qigong derive from their treating the body as a complete system: mind and body. The future of medicine will be an integrative approach of treating both the immediate symptoms of diseases as well as the total person, body and mind.

Large-scale investigations and experiments of the curative effects and functions of TCM and Qigong have been conducted in modern China and elsewhere. Investigators have discovered that the triple heater has many parallels with the lymphatic system. The classical locations of the three heaters are at the groin level, the diaphragm level, and the upper thoracic level, near the heart. This correlates with the major aggregations of lymph nodes in the body. In addition, it has been determined that the lymph nodes are interwoven with neurons. This may suggest that they have an "intelligence" of their own. This investigation into the connection between the immune system and the mind is very exciting. It has been explored in the PBS documentary *Healing and the Mind*.

Modern investigators have also discovered that laughter seems to help heal sickness. How? What happens when one laughs, or practices the sound HEY? Preliminary reports have shown that roaring laughter releases endorphins, a benevolent hormone for the body. Interestingly, the triple heater Healing Sound uses the sound of laughter, HEY. (In the West, *ho* is the sound for laughter, but in China, *hey* is more commonly used.) As one practices the HEY Healing Sound, an overwhelming feeling of joy creates a positive, pervasive warmth in the body. Perhaps, this warmth carries a deep message for the triple heater, the lymphatic system: "Life is fine, life is OK." The Taoists believe that there is a spontaneous healing force for healing and well-being that waits to be ignited. A single laugh may serve as a spark that lights up our spontaneous healing powers.

If you can laugh in the face of serious sickness,
If you can look beyond this earth to the Cosmos,
If you listen very carefully, even in deepest suffering,
Like Milarepa,[1] then you can hear the universe is also laughing.

General Healing Sounds Meditation

Practice the general Healing Sounds meditation as described on pages 48–49. In preparing for the triple heater meditation, you will want to pay special attention to the following. When you rest your hands on the knees with the palms down (or on your thighs with the palms up if you find this more comfortable), very gently tap your ring fingers on the knees to stimulate the triple heater's energy, which runs along the ring finger to the body.

Triple Heater Healing Sound Meditation

The triple heater is our immunolymphatic system. As a warm-up, we will do something that is very popular in China, called Laughing Qigong. Laughter can ignite the spontaneous healing energy and forces within us, for when we laugh, all the internal diaphragms— the pelvic diaphragm, respiratory diaphragm, vocal diaphragm, and cerebral diaphragm—are pumping. This also occurs with crying;

however, Laughing Qigong is more popular. In both cases, the release of positive as well as negative emotions is extremely healthy for the body. In China, they do not have the Marx Brothers—they just sit around and have a belly-shaking laugh. So, place your hands on your knees, inhale, and go "Ho, Ho, Ho." Just laugh like an idiot—don't worry about how you look. Every day, you should laugh for one minute.

To begin, go into your body and visualize your four diaphragms. They are thin and light, like gossamer wings. The pelvic diaphragm is located at the base of your pelvis, the perineum. The respiratory diaphragm is your breathing diaphragm and is located at the bottom of your thoracic chest cavity, below the lungs. The third diaphragm is the vocal diaphragm, a thin membrane stretched in your larynx. Finally, the fourth diaphragm, the cerebral diaphragm (falx cerebri), is a sickle-shaped membrane between the two brain hemispheres. The falx cerebri curves like the dorsal fin of a fish. This diaphragm divides your brain into right and left hemispheres. Try to visualize those four diaphragms, although if you cannot see them, it is OK. Just imagine them.

As you inhale, envision the pelvic diaphragm rising gently like the swelling of a wave. Allow this wave to propel your internal organs upward. Let this serpentine motion radiate up to your respiratory diaphragm. Now gently exhale. Allow the respiratory diaphragm to drop down, letting go of your abdomen, and you will feel a softening of your pelvic diaphragm. As you breathe in naturally, allow the two diaphragms to synchronize their motion. Inhaling like a wave, rise up like a sail filled with air. Exhale and let them drop.

Breathe naturally, taking a few breaths, just like that.

Next we go to the vocal diaphragm, which is located in your larynx. As you inhale, imagine that the vocal diaphragm opens up, stretching open like a resilient rubber band or like a water lily opening. As you exhale, do not contract the rubber band, don't let the flower close, but rather continue to keep the vocal diaphragm open and let it drop down. It is almost a sensation of swallowing a small pill. Continue to experiment and experience the inhaling, allowing the vocal diaphragm to open. Soften the back of your neck and exhale, letting the vocal diaphragm drop down. Now rest for a moment.

Finally, we go to the cerebral diaphragm, which divides the brain into the right and left cerebral hemispheres. Imagine that it is like the dorsal fin of a fish or the sail on a sailboat. As you inhale, allow the cerebral fin to tip slightly forward, toward the front of your body. Make sure you let the back of your neck relax. Moreover, as you exhale, allow the cerebral fin to rock back to its original vertical position. Breathe naturally; experiment and experience a slight rolling, soothing sensation of the head. Inhaling, allow the head to rock forward slightly, and exhaling, allow it to roll back to vertical. Do not let the head drop back further.

Now we will put all four diaphragms together and integrate their movement with our respiration. This is a description of Taoist Qigong reverse breathing. It is not to be taken as a literal, anatomic description of how your breathing apparatus actually moves.

Inhaling, imagine the pelvic and respiratory diaphragms swelling up. As they swell, allow the energy to open the vocal diaphragm, and then the breath goes up and rocks the cerebral fin forward. At the end of the inhalation, pause for a moment to allow all the diaphragms to finish their movement. Exhale. Allow the cerebral fin to rock back slightly, and, letting go of the vocal diaphragm, allow the heart and lungs to rest and the respiratory diaphragm to drop down, finally softening the pelvic diaphragm.

Continue to allow this pumping action of the four diaphragms to synchronize with your breath. Moreover, you may notice that mucus and fluids start to drip down, as well as tears. All those are signs that the pumping action of the diaphragms is working. Feel and experience the wavelike function of these gossamer, winglike structures. Feel their natural motility.

Slowly come back, allowing your eyes to open. Feel a very soft, soothing sensation spreading over the entire body. Yawn if you need to. Stretch your arms out to the side and then down to your knees. Stretch your spine straight up.

Triple Heater Healing Sound Instruction: HEY

Sound Component	Description
Consonant: H	H functions to release stress, stagnation, and phlegm from the lymph system.
Vowel: A	The long *a* vowel combined with the above consonant is like the sound of feed for horses, hay.
Subvocal wind sound: He	He with a breathy, nonvocal sound like a soft sigh of the passing wind. There is a trailing-off of the HEY sound as you come to the end of your breath.

Breath Integrals	Specifics
Tongue	The tongue flattens out to the side with the tip floating freely.
Mouth shape	The lips stretch back as if in a wide grin.

Triple Heater Healing Sound Vocal Instruction

The triple heater sound is HEY. Like all the Healing Sounds, it is divided into three components:

- A consonant sound, which is *h*.
- A vowel sound, which is the long *a*.
- A breath sound, the subvocal wind sound, which is *he*—a kind of sighing, like the sound made by someone who has a high fever, in order to release the excessive heat.

When making the sound, it is important that you keep your mouth open and your tongue stretched flat, with the middle part barely touching the upper palate. It is as if you have a candy in your mouth that you don't want to swallow, but at the same time you want to say, "Hey! That taxi is mine!" So you hold it with your tongue. Please don't try hailing a cab like this—it can be dangerous. This is only an analogy.

Make sure the external shape of your mouth is in an idiotic type of grin, like the Laughing Buddha, Maitreya.

Allow the sound to resonate in your thoracic cavity, behind your sternum (breastbone), causing it to vibrate (see fig. 9.1).

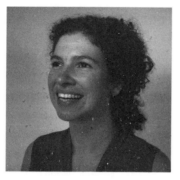

FIGURE 9.1. *HEY*

Triple Heater Healing Sound Movement Instruction

The triple heater movement is simply stretching your arms up, with your palms pushing up to the heavens, as if you are taking a deep yawn.

- *Gather.* Begin with your hands folded one over the other at the Elixir Field (see fig. 9.2).

- *Open.* Inhale, separate your hands slightly out to the side, and unfurl the palms, turning them face up at the Elixir Field. Imagine that your hands become lily pads (see fig. 9.3).

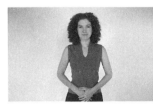

FIGURE 9.2. *Gather*

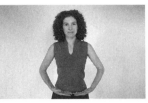

FIGURE 9.3. *Open*

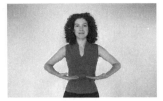

FIGURE 9.4. *Arise*

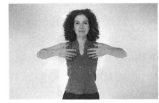

FIGURE 9.5

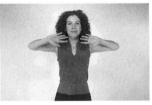

FIGURE 9.6. *Turn Out*

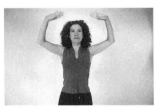

FIGURE 9.7. *Hold Up the Sky*

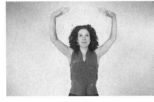

FIGURE 9.8

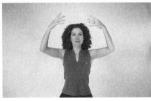

FIGURE 9.9. *Turn In*

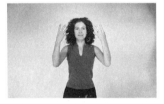

FIGURE 9.10. *Descend*

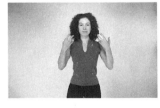

FIGURE 9.11

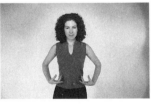

FIGURE 9.12

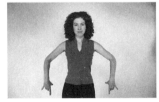

FIGURE 9.13. *Gather*

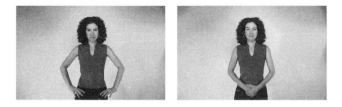

FIGURE 9.14   FIGURE 9.15

- *Arise.* Continuing to inhale, imagine that your palms are like lily pads floating from the bottom of a pond to its surface. Let the palms gently rise from the abdomen to the heart (see figs. 9.4 and 9.5).

- *Turn Out.* Inhale, and turn the palms to face outward. Let the arms separate out to the side a bit (see fig. 9.6). Reminder: As the palms turn outward, let them open away from the body slightly.

- *Hold Up the Sky.* Exhale with the sound HEY. Turn the palms to face the heavens, and reach the palms up as if trying to hold up the sky. Maintain the posture until the full exhalation of HEY is completed (see figs. 9.7 and 9.8). Make sure that you are keeping your shoulders soft, relaxed, and down. Shrug the shoulders a few times; this will help you to drop them. If you feel tension in your shoulders, or pain, do not raise the palms higher than your throat.

- *Turn In.* Inhale, turn your palms in toward yourself, and drop your arms (see fig. 9.9). Feel the warmth from your palms as if they are emanating sunlight.

- *Descend.* Exhale, and let the palms descend along the path from your head, throat, sternum, stomach, and abdomen. Feel as if you are gently washing your face with your palms (see figs. 9.10,

9.11, and 9.12). You may feel a warm, tingling sensation at the different areas of the body as your palms pass over them. This sensation is qi flowing down from the top of the head to the body.

- *Gather.* Inhale, unfurl the hands outward, and let the fingers trace a small semicircle in the air. Overlap the hands at the Elixir Field (see figs. 9.13, 9.14, and 9.15).

- *Repeat.* This completes one cycle of the triple heater Healing Sound Qigong. Repeat the whole cycle three to six times.

Refining the Triple Heater Healing Sound Qigong

The movement of this Qigong is called the Holding Up the Sky Qigong. This posture of Holding Up the Sky is a common theme in Buddhist statues found as lucky charms in many Chinese gift shops. By raising and lowering the palms along the ventral surface of the body, one soothes and harmonizes qi in the three levels of the body. These three levels house the triple heater, with each level corresponding to a particular heater. As you pass your hands in front of your body, imagine joyous warmth radiating from your palms to your abdomen, chest, and face.

Do not arch and curve the spine as you raise the palms upward. Keep the back of the neck relaxed, long, and supple.

Healing Sound Story: Heart Song

Mingli was a professional musician in her fifties. She had recurring breast cancer, and it had started to metastasize throughout her body. I had agreed to teach her Qigong as a complement to her regular cancer therapy. Her doctor and I felt that some form of gentle exercise would help ease her pain from the cancer.

As she walked in, I noticed that her shoulders were slightly hunched forward and her chest was concave, as if it had molded to the shape of her instrument. Her voice was raspy without timbre like a cracked flute. Her face had a chalky pallor.

I asked her for a brief history.

"I am a single mother with an eight-year-old daughter. Eight years ago, when I had breast cancer for the first time, they were able to remove the tumors, and I also received chemotherapy. The cancer was considered in remission. Now, it has recurred and metastasized. My only remaining option is a bone marrow transplant." At the time, this was still an experimental procedure. "Since I have chosen not to do it, my doctor recommended complementary therapies to deal with the pain." I noticed when she mentioned her daughter, Mingli's eyes were downcast.

"So how can I support you?" I asked her.

"I want to learn a daily routine of gentle exercises that can help me to deal with the pain. Even with medications, the pain still keeps me up at night," she replied.

TCM diagnosis showed that Mingli's sickness had penetrated to her bone. Her immune system was very weak, perhaps from the initial chemotherapy and surgery. Her breath was very shallow because of the racking pain.

My basic strategy was twofold: One, free up her breath with the HEY triple heater Healing Sound. Pain, according to TCM principles, is due to a blockage of qi flow. Where there is blockage, pain occurs. By freeing her breath and qi, I hoped to generate a free flow of qi and reduce the pain. Two, teach her the Anti-Cancer Healing Walk, a Qigong walk with a brisk breathing pace.

The Anti-Cancer Healing Walk was discovered by Master Guo Lin. Master Guo Lin had metastasized cancer herself and, after repeated unsuccessful surgeries and chemotherapy, was given six months to live. Only then did she remember what her grandfather, a Taoist, had taught her as a little girl. She started to create her own form of Qigong, the Anti-Cancer Healing Walk, and within a short time her cancer was in spontaneous remission. She has become the grandmother of Qigong therapy and taught millions of cancer patients with great success.[2]

After a month of intensive Qigong and Healing Sounds work, Mingli's health improved. I asked her to keep a daily journal of her practice. It became clear to both of us that after the Qigong practice and Healing Walk, her pain would be relieved for several hours and a sense of joy and well-being would fill her. Her breathing became soft and long. Her voice resounded like a bell. In this period, she felt that her tumors seemed to stabilize. Perhaps she had started on the road to recovery. We redoubled our work in the Qigong sessions for the next three months.

"Can you slow down my recovery? I don't want to lose my disability benefits if I get better too soon. I am not ready to get back to the stress of having to work in the music business," she said one day after our Qigong session.

"What?" I was shocked because she was doing so well. But she was in earnest. I could not imagine an adequate response to her request.

Later, I found out that being a single mother, working and raising her child, was exhausting for Mingli, and she was glad to receive disability. Initially, I was perplexed about her request to slow down her recovery. Was Mingli's fear of getting healthy too quickly derived from her fear of having to jump back into such a hectic life again? Would she rather have cancer than deal with the issues in her life? Later on, I discovered that this is a common pattern. Many patients have subconscious fears of getting well; their sickness allows them to avoid dealing with difficult issues in their life.

After this incident, Mingli's health took a drastic downward turn. We tried several different Qigong approaches, yet the cancer was still spreading. Still, she continued to refuse the bone marrow transplant and decided to go to a special clinic in Mexico. She promised to continue with her Qigong work and to write in her journal.

After a month, I received a three-page letter from Mingli, in shaky and weak handwriting. "Every day I look upon life as a gift from the Divine. I am ready now to accept what my karma brings to life. I have difficulty sleeping because of the pain. The only time that I am free of pain is when I practice the Qigong and Healing Sounds. Only then do I feel a clear sense of wholeness and oneness with everything . . . thank you for giving me this gift of life . . . pray for me. Mingli." It was her last correspondence to me.

Healing and recovery must occur in the context of the whole person, including one's life, one's inner conflicts, and one's body and mind. It is a mistake to treat only the sickness in isolation from the whole person. Perhaps Mingli's cancer was a symptom of her struggle with her life. Or perhaps having a stressful life had contributed to her cancer. In the art of healing, I am constantly humbled by how much I don't know. Mingli's grace and gentleness in the face of suffering has remained a constant inspiration for me to dive deeply into the mystery of life and healing.

Healing Sound Story: Who Should Take Credit?

"Who should take credit?" Mei-mei, a fashion designer, asked her oncologist.

When her X ray and CAT scan showed that her major tumors were reduced in size by 50 percent, she was overjoyed. Four months earlier, Mei-mei was shocked to discover that she had fourth-stage lung cancer, even though she had quit smoking twenty years ago. Dealing with her cancer head on, she embarked on a fully integrative approach of chemotherapy, nutrition, acupuncture, and Qigong.

"Who should take credit for my recovery? Is it my acupuncturist, nutritionist, Qigong practice, or chemotherapy?" she asked the doctor.

"It is you!" the oncologist pointed his finger at her. "Your recovery is remarkable, and I would like to keep a detailed medical file on your progress."

Mei-mei had come to me three months earlier, after discovering that she had advanced lung cancer. Since the major tumor was located close to her aorta, surgery was not an option. Mei-mei was referred to me by her doctor, who was both an acupuncturist and a Western-trained physician.

I recalled the first time she walked in. Her complexion was dark and sallow, and her breathing had a gasping shortness and tightness. Her pulse was tight and hard like the string of an overtuned steel guitar, but her eyes shone with the light of a fighter. This was a good sign— her spirit had not been defeated. Sometimes a person with life-threatening sickness will sink into hopelessness. "How does Qigong support my recovery from cancer?" she asked.

"My professor at the TCM hospital in China taught us this very important truth about healing: The doctor has 25 percent of the solution, the patient has 50 percent, and the rest is up to heaven! I want you to know that the treatment and healing of cancer is teamwork, very much like ants carrying a heavy load. Your doctor, acupuncturist, nutritionist, and I will work together as a team to help your recovery and remission. But you are the central player in this drama.

"First, cancer is not a foreign infection that can be eradicated. Rather, cancer is a complex, multidimensional symptom of various factors: genetic, stress-related, environmental. In Chinese medicine, the proliferation of cancer tumors is due to the weakened state of the triple heater, the immune response system. For you, we will start with freeing up your breathing.

"Now, try to relax and exhale with the Himalayan AH sound. Say it as if, after a hot, sweaty day at work, you have finally slipped into a hot bubble bath. Good. Sense how your chest has started to relax.

"Instinctively, you might be trying to hold your chest as if this will prevent the tumors from spreading. But physically constricting your chest will only restrict your breathing. It will not prevent the tumors from growing or metastasizing. It is important that you bring oxygen into your lungs and bloodstream. Cancer cells are anaerobic, which means that they thrive well without oxygen.

"According to TCM, a major contribution of Qigong as part of an integrative healing strategy is to bring oxygen to the tumors to inhibit their growth. Also the increase in the flow of qi will strengthen your own immune system. Qigong is a perfect complement to your chemotherapy. A daily breathing and Healing Sounds practice will strengthen your body and help repair the damage caused by chemotherapy." Mei-mei started to release the tension she was hold-ing in her chest. She inhaled deeply for the first time since she ar-rived in my office.

"Now, let's begin with the Healing Sound HEY, as if telling your immune system, 'Hey! wake up.' The HEY sound is probably the one that New Yorkers use most often—'Hey, that's my cab!' 'Hey, buddy, wait your turn at the end of the line.'" Mei-mei laughed, and her laughter had a clear ringing sound of hope and inspiration.

For the next several months, I tailored a Qigong program for Mei-mei with the HEY triple heater Healing Sound as her core prac-tice. In my treatment of clients, every person is an individual and re-quires a special regimen for his or her own recovery. "A hundred stomach ulcers require a hundred different prescriptions. That is be-cause there are a hundred unique individuals." This is my Chinese professor's favorite motto.

Three months later, Mei-Mei walked into my office. Her face was radiant. She related her extraordinary tumor shrinkage and how her oncologist gave her credit for her own recovery.

My heart rejoices with feelings of gratitude. I realize that the per-son is truly the star in their own healing story. I am just a cheer-leader, cheering them on.

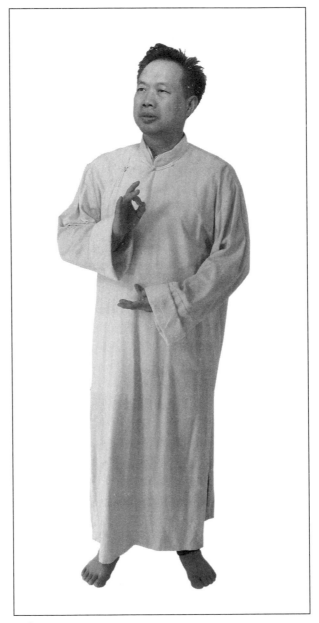

Salute

10

MURMURS OF THE DRAGON

Murmurs of dragons,
Call of lemurs,
"Hey" of hailing cabs,
Each becomes strands of silvery timbres
woven into a single echo,
Booms and surfaces like humpback songs
deep within the sea.

LIKE A MEANDERING STREAM, Taoist practice twists and turns but never cuts a straight line. Such is the way of exploring one's inner terrain. There are no absolutes in Healing Sounds practice. Over the millennia, the Healing Sounds Qigong has evolved into a multitude of branches and styles, each one created in response to the needs of people at that time. In our time of chaos and peace, light and darkness, Healing Sounds Qigong serves as an oasis that cools our overheated organs and quenches our parched spirits.

Do not practice the Healing Sounds Qigong as if trying to fit into uncomfortable foreign clothes. Instead, explore the Healing Sounds; adapt them to your own sensibilities and needs. Treat the Healing Sounds as a gentle lullaby to your organs. Discover aspects of yourself that you have only known from a distance. Be intimate in your practice. Know thyself.

To traverse and explore new terrain, you need a map, a pair of sturdy boots, and a compass—the three hearts of practice.

The Heart of Faith

In exploring any new territory, first we need a map, the heart of faith. Initially, we have to trust that the map is true and can serve as our guide. Likewise, our faith in the healing powers of Six Healing Sounds Qigong lays the foundation of our healing practice. Later, this faith will become faith in our own healing powers, the spontaneous, healing, regenerative forces within us.

My own faith began with my quest for a Taoist master. Though I had studied with several good teachers and martial artists, I felt that I had not yet met my "root" teacher, who would lead me into the inner sanctum of Tao. Eventually, my search led me to an old man living in Chinatown. He had just fled to the United States from Indonesia's Chinese purge. As I entered the one-room apartment, I felt a fluid presence engulf me; standing in the center of a group of students was a man in his late seventies. Without turning, he waved for us to sit on the plastic-covered sofa. By then, I had studied Taiji Quan, Kung Fu, and other martial arts for over ten years. Hmm, let's see what he's got, I said to myself. I had visited many famous masters and had always come away disappointed.

Then he lifted his arm. The spark rippled an electric arc from his toes to his fingertips. His body emerged and dissolved without any discernible motion, like translucent fish swimming in dark water, appearing in one second and vanishing in the next. Appear, vanish, emerge, and dissolve. I was mesmerized by this flickering chimera. Gradually, my cortical lobes glazed over, free of mental debris, pulsating in the wake of his radiance.

He stopped and turned to us. My mother was with me, and by way of introduction she boasted that her son was teaching Taiji in the physical education department at Princeton University. I blushed.

"Would you be so kind as to give us a demonstration?" he asked.

Out of the corner of my eye, I caught a slightly amused glint in his eyes. Since this was the protocol, I had no choice but to perform in front of everyone. Secretly, I was very proud of my Taiji Quan accomplishment.

After twenty minutes, I finished demonstrating my Taiji form. As etiquette required, I went up to ask for his critique.

He mumbled some Chinese words, perhaps just some common polite banter that I couldn't quite catch.

"Mu xi won," he repeated.

The word he said meant "hopeless," and I felt my chest compress as if I were being plunged abruptly into deep water. Images and sounds receded into blue oblivion.

His gaze drilled into me. My mother and everyone else in the room sat in shocked silence. Such brutal frankness was exceptional.

Time felt suspended as if an arrow in slow motion careened straight to my face.

"No hope. I'm sorry. You are too ingrained for me to ever teach you anything new." His voice shot out with a crisp crack. He started to turn away.

I snatched the arrow in the air and replied, "You're right. I am beyond hope of ever learning anything. But I still would like to study with you. So from this point on, I absolve you of all responsibility."

"Good. Then let's go and have some dim sum." He smiled.

I knew then that I had found my root teacher, who would whittle me down to the bone. I surfaced to bright sunlight and blue sky; sound and images returned vivid and clear.

Later, after everyone was seated in the restaurant, I poured a cup of tea. In a traditional Taoist rite of passage, the act of kneeling signifies a surrendering of the ego, and offering tea symbolizes the bonding of teacher and student. For the first time in my life, I went on my knees to offer my teacher a cup of tea. Suddenly, the whole place turned quiet. As he reached for the cup, I noticed that his hands trembled slightly. I knew then that this was my rite of transmission: my first cup of tea to my root teacher must be on my knees.

In Taoist transmission, an initiate must pass a critical test before real teaching can be transmitted. In my case, this occurred in a small apartment in Chinatown. Over the years, I have observed that many students start with great enthusiasm but drop out at the first sign of difficulty. They mistake enthusiasm for faith, but faith must come deep from within one's bones.

For me, having faith meant a complete surrender of ego and pride in my accomplishments. My faith had gained me entrance into the realm of Tao.

In healing, the heart of faith is in believing in your capacity for spontaneous recovery. Everything else—drugs, surgery, medical treatments—is merely supportive of your healing process. In my training in Chinese medicine in China, my professor taught us that the doctor is responsible for only a small part of the patient's recovery. It was a great revelation to learn that my role as a healer is to facilitate the person's healing process.

On the other hand, having the heart of faith does not mean that things will always turn out the way you expect. There is a fine line between faith and delusion. A person under the influence of LSD may truly believe that he can fly. The consequences of acting on such a deluded belief could be fatal. Having faith does not mean one can bring about a specific healing outcome. Do not discredit yourself if your expectation was not fulfilled. Sometimes what we ask and wish for may not turn out to be the way the healing process occurs. Sometimes faith in a person or practice is confused with one's own idealized projection.

My late master certainly did not fulfill my image of a gentle Taoist with a white flowing beard! His ruthless compassion cut me to the bone. During the initial years of serving as his teaching assistant, I often came home in tears. Yet my faith in my own observations and experiences kept me going. I have never blindly followed anyone without verification from my own experience.

As you practice the Healing Sounds, your own experiences will confirm your faith in their healing effects. Study and practice the Healing Sounds with an open sense of discovery. You will build a strong foundation for subsequent Qigong practices.

Having faith is only the first step, however. Collecting maps of a place is not the same as going there. Armed with the map, now you are ready to plunge into the art of practice.

The Heart of Perseverance

The heart of perseverance is like a good pair of boots. It allows you to hike a long, difficult journey. Likewise, the heart of perseverance will support your practicing diligently. A renowned composer once told me that spiritual practice means actually doing it, not just accumulating intellectual knowledge. As a composer, he knows instinctively that just reading about music will not improve his ability to play the piano. Even with his busy schedule, he has maintained his Qigong practice every single day from his first lesson. That was several years ago! Persevering in one's daily practice is fraught with difficulty and obstruction. Sometimes, you may feel as if you are swimming against the current. Life keeps throwing obstacles in the path of your practice. Actually, you are confronting your old habits and conditionings. Until you can establish the Healing Sounds as part of your daily life, try to practice in a "needlepoint" way, which is to thread a small amount of practice between your other activities. For example, while waiting for a train, quietly practice the spleen Healing Sound of FU to soothe the anxiety of waiting. Or before lunch, just sit back a moment to say the heart HO sound and be glad of having food to eat. However, do not do the Healing Sounds while you are driving a car or operating any dangerous equipment that requires total concentration.

Daily practice means always having energy in reserve. Do not practice to the brink of utter exhaustion. Rather, practice to the point of feeling good. Stop when you feel you could practice for just another five minutes—that is a good time to finish. Practicing to the point of exhaustion will only risk physical and mental damage. Your organs will overheat, and minute particles and waste will overwhelm your bloodstream.

After having gone through the Six Healing Sounds, choose one or two sounds, or a combination of sounds, as your daily routine. The Healing Sounds are such benevolent Qigong that any combination will offer health benefits. Of course, it is best to do the full Six Healing Sounds.

Nevertheless, the Healing Sounds should not serve as a replacement for your prescribed therapy or medicine. Heart patients should always continue to take their heart medicine even as they do the Healing Sounds. The Healing Sounds are wonderful complementary practices for health and healing.

Having firmly rooted Healing Sounds practice in your daily life, you will notice in subtle ways that your day will be more peaceful and happy. In some rare cases, however, a student may experience slight discomfort while practicing the Healing Sounds, such as dizziness, shortness of breath, spontaneous shaking, or mild headaches. In these cases, stop practicing and seek out a physician to verify whether you are suffering from any disorder or sickness.

If, after a thorough checkup, the doctor gives you a clean bill of health, then resume the Healing Sounds practice. In this case, the Healing Sounds may have triggered a release of internal qi sickness that caused the discomfort. Reduce the range of motion and check whether you are straining yourself. Soften the Healing Sounds or even do just the silent subvocal sounds without the vowel. In time, the symptom will ease and vanish.

In rare cases, the discomfort may persist even after you have followed this protocol. Then you must seek out a competent Qigong master to modify your Qigong practice.

The heart of perseverance is symbolized by the water in the Grand Canyon: no matter how obstructed the river becomes, the water continues to flow toward the sea. The water in its eternal patience has carved the deep gorges. Similarly, with the heart of perseverance, you can wear away chronic sickness in minute increments.

The Heart of Wisdom

To cultivate awareness is the heart of wisdom. Having the heart of Wisdom is like having a compass that guides us on our journey. This metaphysical compass will always point to one direction—awareness. How often do we pay attention to the way we sit, stand, or sleep? How often do we pay attention to our life? To be aware is to pay attention to actions, movement, speech, and consciousness. Awareness is a ripple that expands to encompass all things.

For example, during standing practice, many students tilt their body slightly forward, without realizing that their weight is out of balance. Only by looking at their reflection in the mirror will they discover that they are off balance. The six physical and inner pairings explained in chapter 3 are basic self awareness tools to assess one's alignment and balance.

Six Healing Sounds Qigong cultivates awareness through sound and movement. This dynamic awareness enables us to sense and feel the quality of sounds and movements. Hence, such sensing improves and refines our Qigong practice. Otherwise, the Healing Sounds practice can become just another boring exercise routine. The intention and awareness in the practice of Qigong spontaneously directs the healing power to even hidden sickness. Clear intent and vivid awareness are the sparks that ignite spontaneous healing.

Therefore, the final aspect of Taoist practice is cultivating the heart of wisdom. Actions without awareness are like rowing in the dark with the boat still anchored. Our movements are often moored by the anchor of habitual tensions, which reduce the Qigong's effectiveness. Only with awareness can we correct and remove those habitual tensions.

In Taoist initiation, disciples are empowered by the touch of the master's finger at their celestial eye—the space between the eyebrows. This symbolizes the opening of their wisdom eye. After this, the adepts can steer a clear course in their Taoist practice. The difference between being aware and being unaware is like the difference between walking with eyes wide open or stumbling with eyes shut tight. Open your inner eyes, and the world unfolds in your palms. Trees, flowers, and your own children can be your own teachers as well. When you are receptive, a strand of cloud in the evening sky expounds the profound truth of awakening. Then faith and perseverance flow into one, wisdom.

Q: What is the difference between your Healing Sounds and other schools of Healing Sounds?

A: The difference is emphasis. Other styles emphasize the internal image of smiling to the organs, while we integrate internal visualization, meditation, sound, and movement to stimulate the qi flow. There is no conflict between the two practices, just a difference in focus.

Q: If I have a mental disorder, what sound should I practice?

A: Here lies the tricky part of self-diagnosis. I have heard my clients diagnose their own sickness, and usually their conclusions and solutions run counter to most established TCM principles. It takes extensive training and experience to make a correct diagnosis of sickness based on external symptoms and other subtle signs. The Six Healing Sounds, as they are presented here, are not meant to correspond to specific diseases. It is dangerous to prescribe for one's own sickness or to use the general label of "mental disorder." The best strategy is to practice all of the Six Healing Sounds gently. It is misleading to think that HO—the heart Healing Sound—alone will heal mental disorders, even though the heart as an organ functions as part of the nervous system.

Q: Can I practice if I am pregnant?

A: Yes. The Healing Sounds are very soothing for the fetus. You will discover that daily practice will help ease some of the stress of pregnancy. Of course, you should be under the care of a physician.

Q: Can I create my own Healing Sounds?

A: Ancient Taoist masters who had great depth of insight into the human energetic pathways created the Six Healing Sounds. Unless you are an accomplished Taoist master, your own personal Healing Sound may not be so well rounded and universal. Recently, a professor created his own form of meditation by having his college students chant "Me, Me, Me. . . ." Obviously, they failed to reach a state of tranquillity. However, it is possible that for your own personal use, you will discover that doing certain Healing Sounds with a slight variation may produce a greater sense of well-being. Then by all means continue to practice your personal Healing Sounds.

Q: Can I teach the heart Healing Sound to my grandfather who has just had a heart attack?

A: No. A person who has just suffered a serious trauma should recover his strength first. Only when his doctor allows for gentle exercises or physical therapy should you begin teaching him the Healing Sound. Starting with the meditation that accompanies the Healing Sound is a gentle way to help recovery. Sometimes acting on our impulse to help our loved ones without a clear understanding of the situation may actually harm them.

Q: I am a massage therapist; can I teach the Healing Sounds to my clients?

A: The Healing Sounds can support the body to recover its spontaneous self-healing power. Showing the Healing Sounds to your clients after treatment is a wonderful way of empowering their own self-healing. It is my own experience of studying with many traditional Chinese doctors that they all give their patients "homework" to speed up their recovery. Of course, it is even better if you can give them this book as a further support for their healing.

Q: Can I integrate the Healing Sounds Qigong with yoga or other spiritual practices?

A: Yes. The Taoist Healing Sounds overlap with the yogic mantra system. Integrating the Healing Sounds in the beginning of your yogic or other spiritual practice is like pouring cream into your coffee— it will make your other practice smooth and light. Many of my students are yoga teachers who benefit greatly from integrating Qigong into their daily practice.

Q: I have heard that Qigong can cure cancer. Can the Healing Sounds Qigong heal cancer?

A: It is true that in China there is clinical data to support Qigong practices causing spontaneous remission in cancer patients. At this point, those clinical trials are not accepted in the West because they lacked control groups, which in this case would be a group of cancer patients who were instructed to practice a phony kind of made-up Qigong. This runs counter to Chinese ethical standards. No Qigong master would willingly teach a very sick person phony Qigong in the name of scientific research.

Since cancer is a hydra with many heads, no simple treatment will cause an effective remission. The Six Healing Sounds Qigong is designed to improve one's general health and well-being; it is not set up as a specific cancer treatment. However, it could serve as a complementary practice alongside the established cancer treatment protocols. The correct practice of the Healing Sounds will improve overall circulation and respiration. Therefore, it indirectly helps the body to recover from and maximize the benefits of cancer treatment.

This principle of integrative and complementary medicine fits very well with the Qigong therapeutic approach of using the Six Healing Sounds.

Q: Are there any other resources to guide my Healing Sounds practices?

A: Yes. If you have access to the Internet you can log on to the Dantao Web site at *www.dantao.com,* where you will find monthly articles and related resources on the general field of Qigong and Taiji Quan.

Q: I experienced some discomfort during my Six Healing Sounds Qigong practice. Should I stop doing Qigong completely, or just continue and ignore the discomfort?

A: If you experience any pain or discomfort, immediately stop the exercise and consult a physician. Pain and discomfort are often an indication that you have overstrained your body. The postures and movements must be altered to correct any excessive physical strain. Remember, pain or discomfort is an indication that something is wrong—it is a message. Please see appendix B for additional protocols for dealing with uncommon sensations or experiences during Qigong practice.

APPENDIX B

Protocols for Difficulties in Practicing the Healing Sounds

The following are general guidelines for when you experience un-usual symptoms during Qigong practice. This information is given as a precautionary measure for extreme cases. Most people will not notice any unusual reactions to the Healing Sounds.

Symptom	Diagnosis	Practice
Discomfort	Consult a physician to verify the cause of discomfort.	Resume practice of Healing Sound if given medical clearance. Try a reduced range of motion and shorter duration.
Internal vision of light, images, or symbols	Consult a physician. If no physical cause is discovered and there is no previous trauma to the eyes or brain, then this could be a sign that the qi is opening the channel and meridians in your brain.	Resume practice if given medical clearance. Do not fixate on the visions or take them for reality. Again, the vision is a manifestation of qi. It will dissolve after continued practice.

Symptom	Diagnosis	Practice
Sensation of excessive heat that seems to run down different parts of the body	Consult a physician. This is a common sign of blood and qi flowing freely.	Resume practice if given medical clearance. Do not fixate on the sensation of the heat, and eventually it will be less pronounced. With continued practice, a pervasive soothing warmth envelops one's whole body.
Persistent tingling sensation in the fingertips, hands, or other parts of the body, during and after Qigong practice	Consult a physician to verify whether there is pinching of nerves. If no pinching of nerves is found, it could be that qi is opening a blockage in the energy channels of that particular part of the body.	If there is pinching of nerves, consult a physician for the best course of action. Verify with the doctor whether the Qigong practice as indicated in this book is beneficial for you. Reduce the range of motion; do less and change your posture to see if it relieves the sensations. With continuous practice, once the energy channels are open, the tingling will dissipate completely.
Internal hearing of sounds and voices	Consult a physician. If the symptom is not due to any psychological sickness or psychotropic drugs, this may be an echo of the Healing Sounds, a common occurrence.	Resume practice if given medical clearance. In many instances, chanting the Healing Sound in a group setting will produce these phenomena; the yogis called this the cosmic harmonics. Do not pay any attention to the sound; gradually it will either dissipate or become just part of your practice.

Symptom	Diagnosis	Practice
Dizziness or headache	Consult a physician. If no physical cause is found, this could be a result of the increased flow of oxygen to your brain.	Resume practice if given medical clearance. Sometimes this is caused by hyperventilation. You need to shorten the length of chanting of the Healing Sound. Try to say the sound in a more relaxed manner without excessive effort.
Shaking and spontaneous movement during Qigong practice	Consult a physician to verify the cause of shaking and spontaneous movements. In Taoist diagnosis, spontaneous movement is due to excessive liver qi spilling into the muscle and ligament systems of the body.	Resume practice if given medical clearance. Reduce your focus during the practice. Relax your gaze and concentration. Make sure your breathing is soft and at ease.

Do not be frightened by the above information. Most people will not experience these symptoms. However, if you do feel some of these sensations, the most important thing is to remain calm, consult your physician as indicated, and when you're cleared to practice, don't fixate on the sensation.

$$NOTES$$

SONG OF THE SHAMANS

1. *The Jade Maiden Canon on Tantric Healing* is a controversial book that is attributed to the Yellow Emperor. It was most likely written much later than 200 B.C.E., more likely in the era of 500 C.E.

2. Translation from Chuang Tzu, *Inner Chapter of Chuang Tzu* (Beijing, China: Zhong Hua Press, 1982), p. 43.

3. Translated from Hui Szu, *Ta Ch'eng Chih Kuan* (Mahayana samatha-vipassana) (Beijing, China: China Buddhist Association Press, 1968), p. 1078.

4. Translated from Zhen Jiu Dai Chen, *The Complete Work on Acupuncture and Moxabustion* (Beijing, China: People's Health Ministry Press, 1984), p. 1268.

5. From the *Suragama Sutra* (Beijing, China: China Buddhist Association Press, 1974), p. 346. For an English translation of the sutra, see Charles Luk, *The Secret of Chinese Meditation* (York Beach, Maine: Samuel Weiser, Inc., 1964), p. 32.

CHAPTER 2. *Macrocosm and Microcosm:*
Taoist Concepts of Health and Therapeutics

1. *New Compilation of Chinese Medicine Essential Principles,* (Beijing, China: People's Ministry of Health Press, 1974), p. 174.

2. In Arthurian legend, Merlin is a magician who assisted King

Arthur in assembling his kingdom. Being an alchemist, Merlin grows in the opposite direction from most people—he grows younger rather than older. A wonderful tale of Merlin and the king is told by T. H. White in *The Sword in the Stone* (New York: Philomel Books, 1993).

CHAPTER 3. *Principles of Core Harmonics*

1. Numen in Chinese is *shen*, which has the broad meaning of spirit, mind, consciousness, and psyche. Sexual essence in Chinese is *jing*, which has the inclusive meaning of life force, libido, sperm, and sex hormones.
2. The Ouroboros is an ancient alchemical symbol: a serpent with its tail in its mouth, continuously devouring itself and being re-born from itself. The Ouroboros expresses the unity of all things; it is the cycle of material and spiritual, body and mind, which never disappear but perpetually change form in an eternal cycle of destruction and re-creation. The Ouroboros forms the archaic Chinese word *shen*, a circular star constellation. This became the fifth hour of the lunar daily clock.

CHAPTER 6. *Spleen: The Mother Earth*

1. Tate, Seeley, and Stephens, *Understanding the Human Body* (St. Louis, Missouri: Mosby-Year Book, Inc., 1994), p. 266.

CHAPTER 7. *Lungs: The Knights in Shining Armor*

1. The energy field pattern has been document by special photography that can film infrared light. In one photograph, a leaf energy pattern was clearly visible on the plant although the leaf had been cut off. John Iovine, *Kirlian Photography* (N.Y.: McGraw Hill, 1994).

CHAPTER 8. *Kidneys: Fire and Water*

1. This is a Chinese prescription for very specific symptoms. Readers who you have similar symptoms should have a thorough medical examination. Fainting can be a sign of serious illness.

CHAPTER 9. *Triple Heater: The Organic Furnace*

1. Milarepa was a Tibetan Buddhist saint of great wisdom who is often represented in statues and paintings with one palm to his ear, listening to the sound of universal laughter.
2. Guo Lin, *A New Approach to Qigong Therapy for Cancer Healing* (Beijing, China: Guo Lin Qigong Association Press, 1974).